Genitourinary
Tuberculosis

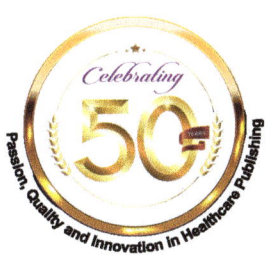

Genitourinary Tuberculosis

Editors

Ganesh Gopalakrishnan MS MCh Urology
Ex HOD, CMC Vellore
Consultant Urologist
Vedanayagam Hospital
Coimbatore, Tamil Nadu, India

Sujata Patwardhan MS MCh Urology
Professor and Head
Department of Urology
Seth GS Medical College and KEM Hospital
Mumbai, Maharashtra, India

Foreword
P Venugopal

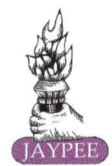

JAYPEE BROTHERS MEDICAL PUBLISHERS
The Health Sciences Publisher
New Delhi | London

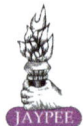 **Jaypee Brothers Medical Publishers (P) Ltd**

Headquarters
Jaypee Brothers Medical Publishers (P) Ltd
4838/24, Ansari Road, Daryaganj
New Delhi 110 002, India
Phone: +91-11-43574357
Fax: +91-11-43574314
Email: jaypee@jaypeebrothers.com

Overseas Offices
J.P. Medical Ltd
83 Victoria Street, London
SW1H 0HW (UK)
Phone: +44 20 3170 8910
Fax: +44 (0)20 3008 6180
Email: info@jpmedpub.com

Website: www.jaypeebrothers.com
Website: www.jaypeedigital.com

© 2020, Jaypee Brothers Medical Publishers

The views and opinions expressed in this book are solely those of the original contributor(s)/author(s) and do not necessarily represent those of editor(s) of the book.

All rights reserved. No part of this publication may be reproduced, stored or transmitted in any form or by any means, electronic, mechanical, photocopying, recording or otherwise, without the prior permission in writing of the publishers.

All brand names and product names used in this book are trade names, service marks, trademarks or registered trademarks of their respective owners. The publisher is not associated with any product or vendor mentioned in this book.

Medical knowledge and practice change constantly. This book is designed to provide accurate, authoritative information about the subject matter in question. However, readers are advised to check the most current information available on procedures included and check information from the manufacturer of each product to be administered, to verify the recommended dose, formula, method and duration of administration, adverse effects and contraindications. It is the responsibility of the practitioner to take all appropriate safety precautions. Neither the publisher nor the author(s)/editor(s) assume any liability for any injury and/or damage to persons or property arising from or related to use of material in this book.

This book is sold on the understanding that the publisher is not engaged in providing professional medical services. If such advice or services are required, the services of a competent medical professional should be sought.

Every effort has been made where necessary to contact holders of copyright to obtain permission to reproduce copyright material. If any have been inadvertently overlooked, the publisher will be pleased to make the necessary arrangements at the first opportunity. The **CD/DVD-ROM** (if any) provided in the sealed envelope with this book is complimentary and free of cost. **Not meant for sale.**

Inquiries for bulk sales may be solicited at: jaypee@jaypeebrothers.com

Genitourinary Tuberculosis / *Ganesh Gopalakrishnan, Sujata Patwardhan*

First Edition: **2020**

ISBN: 978-93-89776-68-3

Printed at:

CONTRIBUTORS

Editors

Ganesh Gopalakrishnan MS MCh Urology
Ex HOD, CMC Vellore
Consultant Urologist
Vedanayagam Hospital
Coimbatore, Tamil Nadu, India

Sujata Patwardhan MS MCh Urology
Professor and Head
Department of Urology
Seth GS Medical College and KEM Hospital
Mumbai, Maharashtra, India

Co-Editors

Umesh Shelke MS MCh Urology
Consultant Urologist
Wockhardt Hospital
Nagpur, Maharashtra, India

Ajit Sawant MCh Urology
Professor and HOD
Department of Urology
Lokmanya Tilak Medical
College and Hospital, Sion
Mumbai, Maharashtra, India

Rishikesh Velhal MS MCh Urology
Assistant Professor
Department of Urology
KEM Hospital
Mumbai, Maharashtra, India

Nikhar Jain MS
Senior Resident Urology, 2017
Admission for MCh Urology
KEM Hospital
Mumbai, Maharashtra, India

Rupali Sable MD
Assistant Professor
Department of PSM
KEM Hospital
Mumbai, Maharashtra, India

Yash Pamecha MS MCh Urology
Senior Registrar
Department of Urology
KEM Hospital
Mumbai, Maharashtra, India

Contributing Authors

Anila Abraham Kurien MD Pathology
Consultant Pathologist
Renopath Centre for Renal and
Urological Pathology
Chennai, Tamil Nadu, India

Camilla Rodrigues MD Microbiology
Consultant Microbiologist and
Chairperson Infection Control Committee
PD Hinduja Hospital
Mahim, Mumbai, Maharashtra, India

Anuj Deep Dangi MS Mch Urology
Professor, Department of Urology
CMC Vellore
Tamil Nadu, India

Ganesh Gopalakrishnan MS MCh Urology
Ex HOD, CMC Vellore
Consultant Urologist, Vedanayagam Hospital
Coimbatore, Tamil Nadu, India

Narendra Sutar MBBS
District TB Officer
Department of Tuberculosis
MCGM
Mumbai, Maharashtra, India

Nitin Kekre MS Mch Urology
Professor
Department of Urology
CMC Vellore
Tamil Nadu, India

S Boopathy Vijayaraghavan MD Radiology
Consultant Radiologist
Sonoscan Centre Coimbatore
Tamil Nadu, India

Sujata Patwardhan MS MCh Urology
Professor and Head
Department of Urology
Seth GS Medical College and KEM Hospital
Mumbai, Maharashtra, India

Suleman Merchant MD Radiology
Ex Professor and Head of Department
Radiology, LTMG Sion Hospital
Ex Dean LTM Medical College and
LTMG Sion Hospital
Mumbai, Maharashtra, India

Sunil D Khaparde MD PhD FIAP FIPHA
Advisor, Public Health SPL, PHO
Ministry of Health and Family Welfare
Government of India
Mumbai, Maharashtra, India

Yash Pamecha MS MCh Urology
Senior Registrar
Department of Urology
KEM Hospital
Mumbai, Maharashtra, India

FOREWORD

Tuberculosis continues to be a *public health problem* in most countries around the globe and it is more so in India.

Tuberculosis of urinary and genital organs is ancient but it continues to remain as an unsolved problem. Clinical features are flexible and genitourinary tuberculosis (GUTB) presentations are so varied that it can mimic many other conditions. Approximate 8,000 articles are available in the literature but there is probably no study encompassing all aspects of the disease. Most of them are quite superficial addressing some aspect of this disease. Hence to compile all aspects of the disease, even as a textbook, is well-nigh impossible.

The main issue attached to the problem is that delay in diagnosis and proper initiation of early treatment very often result in progress of disease leading to eventual renal functional deterioration. In many, the old statement that "Bladder is the Vocal cord of Kidney" is true as many present with varying bladder symptoms. This adds to the confusion as to the diagnosis of urinary tuberculosis.

The sequelae following proper treatment resulting in functional changes have to be borne in mind and need very frequent follow-ups and evaluation even after commencing treatment.

It has been noticed that though there are several diagnostic tests now available, the overall efficacy of detecting GUTB is being questioned by some. Hence, the question asked is whether one will have to wait for the results of diagnostic tests prior to initiation of treatment by drugs. Can the treatment be initiated on high index of suspicion? Professor HS Bhat (Doyen of Urology in India) often used to mention that "Urologists should be able to sniff GUTB". According to him, even diagnosing by bacteriological tests and radiology is often too late. This view is now being questioned by many and mentions that the condition should be diagnosed beyond doubt to commence treatment.

Ganesh and Sujata have to be complemented for bringing out this book on time covering most aspects that we have to know and understand. The 26 cases illustrated provide more than adequate representation on all aspects of GUTB that we frequently encounter. Such a compiling adds considerable value for the book.

I am sure this book is a must read for all urologists across the globe and even for those countries where GUTB may not be under much consideration.

P Venugopal MBBS MS MCh (Urology)
Retired Professor Urology, KMC
Manipal, Karnataka, India

PREFACE

India accounts for 23% of the global burden of tuberculosis. In 2014 of a total of 9.6 million cases worldwide, 2.2 million cases of tuberculosis were estimated to have occurred in India. Renal tuberculosis is the most common site of extrapulmonary genitourinary tuberculosis (GUTB) comprising of 20% of all extrapulmonary tuberculosis (EPTB).

In 2014, the Central TB Division and Directorate General of Health Services of the Ministry of Health and Family Welfare, Government of India, recognized the need to develop evidence-informed guidelines for EPTB. This was aimed to run concurrently with those for pulmonary tuberculosis from the Revised National TB Control Programme (RNTCP). Unfortunately, evidence-based guidelines for treatment of GUTB are lacking. Should a 6-month regimen be sufficient or should it be 9 months.

While there are individual chapters in various textbooks relating to different aspects of GUTB, a single book devoted to renal tuberculosis is lacking. We, the editors felt that the vast experience in our country by individual physicians should be collated in a comprehensive book which would help urologists enhance their knowledge and also serve to manage our patients effectively.

This has been possible only because of the commitment of the authors who themselves have felt such a need and the untiring efforts of Drs Umesh Shelke and Yash Pamecha both ex-residents of the Urology Department, KEM Hospital, Mumbai.

Ganesh Gopalakrishnan
Sujata Patwardhan

ACKNOWLEDGMENTS

We would like to thank Drs Umesh Shelke, Yash Pamecha, Rishikesh Velhal, Nikhar Jain, ex and present staff of the Department of Urology, KEM Hospital, Mumbai for their untiring effort. We would like to especially appreciate Dr Rupali Sable, Department of Preventive and Social Medicine, KEM Hospital, for providing us the source material for this publication.

Last but not the least, we would like to thank Mr Padmanabhan and his team from Dr Reddy's Laboratories for supporting this venture.

We also want to acknowledge the sincere efforts and enthusiasm of Shri Jitendar P Vij, Mr Sabarish Menon, Dr Richa Saxena, Dr Nidhi Sood and their team from Jaypee Brothers Medical Publishers (P) Ltd for carrying out the process of publication swiftly and completing the book in short span of time.

ABBREVIATIONS

AKT	Anti-Kock treatment
BDQ	Bedaquiline
C-DST	Culture and drug susceptibility testing
c/o	Complaint of
CAT 1	Category 1
CBNAAT	Cartridges based nucleic acid amplification test
CSIC	Clean self intermittent catheterization
CT	Computed tomography
DDR-TBC	District Drug Resistant Tuberculosis Centre
DMC	Designated Microscopy Centre
DM	Diabetes mellitus
DR-TB	Drug-resistant tuberculosis
DST	Drug Susceptibility Testing
DVDMS	Drug Vaccine Distribution Management System
e/o	Evidence of
EPDR-TB	Extrapulmonary drug-resistant tuberculosis
EP	Extrapulmonary
EPTB	Extrapulmonary tuberculosis
ESRD	End-stage renal disease
FL-LPA	First line probe assay
GUTB	Genitourinary tuberculosis
h/o	History of
HIV	Human immunodeficiency syndrome
IVP	Intravenous pyelography
k/c/o	Known complaint of
LPA	Line probe assay
LUTS	Lower urinary tract symptoms
MDR-TB	Multidrug resistant tuberculosis
MRI	Magnetic resonance imaging
MR-TB	Mono-resistant tuberculosis
PDR-TB	Poly-drug resistant tuberculosis
PMDT	Programmatic management of drug-resistant tuberculosis
PTB	Pulmonary tuberculosis
r/o	Resident of
RNTCP	Revised National Tuberculosis Control Program
RRTB	Rifampicin-resistant tuberculosis
s/o	suggestive of
TBC	Tuberculosis contact
TB	Tuberculosis
WHO	World Health Organization
XDR-TB	Extensively drug-resistant tuberculosis

CONTENTS

1. Tuberculosis Epidemiology in India   1
   Sunil D Khaparde

2. Excerpts from Guidelines on Management of
   Drug-resistant Tuberculosis   14
   Sujata Patwardhan, Narendra Sutar

3. Pathology of Tuberculosis in the Genitourinary Tract   36
   Anila Abraham Kurien

4. Microbiology of Today's Relevance   45
   Camilla Rodrigues, Yash Pamecha

5. Imaging Studies in Genitourinary Tuberculosis   52
   Suleman Merchant, Sujata Patwardhan

6. Sonographic Features of Urinary Tuberculosis   60
   S Boopathy Vijayaraghavan

7. Outline of Medical and Surgical Management   92
   Sujata Patwardhan

8. Surgery Outcomes   98
   Nitin Kekre, Anuj Deep Dangi

9. Interesting Cases   112
   Ganesh Gopalakrishnan, Sujata Patwardhan, Ajit Sawant, Umesh Shelke
   - Case 1 112
   - Case 2 114
   - Case 3 118
   - Case 4 121
   - Case 5 123
   - Case 6 126
   - Case 7 129
   - Case 8 130
   - Case 9 133
   - Case 10 136
   - Case 11 138
   - Case 12 140
   - Case 13 143

Case 14 145
Case 15 147
Case 16 151
Case 17 153
Case 18 155
Case 19 159
Case 20 161
Case 21 163
Case 22 165
Case 23 179
Case 24 182
Case 25 185
Case 26 186

Index *189*

CHAPTER 1

Tuberculosis Epidemiology in India

Sunil D Khaparde

Each year, in India, an estimated 28 lacs people develop tuberculosis (TB) disease and approximately 4.8 lacs people die from TB— World Health Organization's (WHO's) Global Report 2017.

A study of mortality in India has estimated that TB is among the top four causes of death between the ages of 30 and 69 years, with an impact similar to cancer. The socioeconomic impact of TB in India is devastating and India continues to incur huge costs due to TB amounting to nearly US$ 350 billion between 2006 and 2015.

India continues to have the highest TB burden though the epidemic is on the decline. The incidence of TB, human immunodeficiency virus (HIV) and TB (5%), and drug-resistant tuberculosis (DR-TB) varies from region to region. The urban areas have lower prevalence of TB with a higher annual risk of tuberculous infection (ARTI) and vice versa.

This is the reason why different approaches are necessary to tackle the problem. The National TB Programme of India (NTP) was initiated in 1962 and was originally designed for domiciliary treatment, using self-administered standard drug regimens. NTP had created an extensive infrastructure for TB control with a network of > 446 district TB centers, 330 TB clinics and > 47,600 TB beds. The NTP had also raised awareness of TB and TB treatment facilities, and had succeeded in placing > 1.3 million patients on treatment annually.

The problems are HIV-AIDS epidemic and the spread of multidrug-resistant (MDR) TB were threatening to further worsen in the situation.

Inadequate funding, an over reliance on X-ray for diagnosis, had frequent interrupted supplies of drug, and low rates of treatment completion. The government decided to give new thrust to TB control activities by revitalizing the NTP with assistance from international agencies in 1993. Revised National TB Control Programme (RNTCP) was piloted in a population of 2.4 million of five states. This was later expanded to cover 13 million people by 1995 and 20 million by 1996.

In 1997, the RNTCP was launched as national program with the plan to scale up in phased manner. It adopted the internationally recommended directly observed treatment short-course (DOTS) strategy, as the systematic and cost-effective approach to revitalize the TB control program in India.

The program is credited with saving 3.5 million lives and initiation of 19 million patients.

Emboldened by its achievements, the program in 12th Five Year Plan (2012–2017) has articulated a vision of universal access to TB care with the following objectives: (i) To achieve 90% notification rate for all cases; (ii) to achieve 90% success rate for all new and 85% for retreatment cases; (iii) to significantly improve the successful outcomes of treatment of DR-TB cases; (iv) to achieve decreased morbidity and mortality of HIV-associated TB; and (v) to improve outcomes of TB care in the private sector.

National AIDS Control Programme and RNTCP have started a "National Framework of Joint TB/HIV Collaborative Activities" by engaging the private sector of medical care and professional bodies like Indian Medical Association (IMA). A case-based web-based platform "Nikshay" in 2012 has now been scaled up nationally.

STANDARDS FOR TB CARE IN INDIA (STCI)

The private sector holds a factual predominance of healthcare service delivery in India. There is very little information about TB patients from the private sector which is available to the program and little is known about their quality of treatment, including treatment outcomes.

"The National Strategic Plan (NSP) for TB Elimination (2017–2025) is a statement of commitment to eliminate TB by 2025 by the Ministry of Health and Family Welfare, Government of India." The NSP builds on the success and learnings of the last NSP and encapsulates the bold and innovative steps required to eliminate TB in India. It is in line with other health sector strategies and global efforts, such as the National Health Policy 2015, WHO's End TB strategy, and the sustainable development goals (SDGs) of the United Nations (UN). It proposes bold strategies with commensurate resources to rapidly decline TB incidence and mortality in India by 2025, 5 years ahead of the global End TB targets and SDGs. The NSP 2017–2025 aims to notify 260 lacs TB patients in 8 years including public and private sector.

In the 12th Plan period (2012–2017), RNTCP was implemented under the umbrella of the National Health Mission (NHM).[1] The same is proposed to be continued in the current plan period. The program has successfully achieved the Millennium Development Goal for incidence and prevalence of TB.
- The incidence of TB has come down from 289 per lac population in 2000 to 217 per lac (58%) population in 2015.
- The mortality from TB has reduced from 56 in 2000 to 36 per lac (28%) population in 2015.

However, India still accounts for an estimated 27% of the global incident TB cases (28 lacs) and 27% of the global MDR-TB cases (1.3 lacs).

The activities under the program currently ongoing would be continued and specific activities/focus areas proposed are as under:
- Increase participation of private sector TB care provider: TB notification has increased substantially in these pilot areas with providing free TB diagnostics and drugs provided either directly by state public health system or through nongovernmental organizations (NGOs) or agencies supporting the states. It is also proposed to provide incentives to the private sector TB care provider through direct beneficiary transfer to promote TB case notification, ensure treatment adherence, and treatment completion.
- Intensified TB control activities in high priority districts: Active case finding (ACF) or intensive case finding (ICF) activity is an activity with the primary objective of detecting TB cases early. Clinically, socially, and occupationally vulnerable populations

are targeted by screening for TB symptoms, to conduct sputum examination of symptomatic using a high sensitive and specific tool in the field and to find and treat additional infectious TB patients.
- Providing incentive to prevent catastrophic expenditure to the TB patients and their families due to TB and for nutritional support: This interaction is particularly important in the Indian context where poverty and undernutrition coexist with a large burden of tuberculosis. It is proposed to launch a scheme to provide a monthly cash incentive for every TB patient through direct beneficiary transfer.
- Deploy a world-class national surveillance and tracking system for TB patients: Nikshay will be enhanced to establish comprehensive real time TB surveillance system. Information and communication technology (ICT) platform with handheld ICT devises for health staff, 250 seats call centers, adherence mechanisms through 99-DOTS, SMS reminders and other ICT-based platforms are proposed with corresponding HR and maintenance capacity.

Government of India envisages TB control as one of the key priority activities and is committed to an aspirational target of achieving this ahead of schedule—by the year 2025.
- India has developed NSP for TB in India. The NSP for TB elimination in India has essentially 4 pillars to address the major challenges for TB control, namely "Detect, Treat, Build and Prevent".
- Priority for TB control in India are:
  ○ The first priority is "reaching the unreached". We have to ensure access to care for some vulnerable populations such as tribals, people in urban slums, etc.
- 25% of the budget is earmarked for patients managed in the private sector. This include free diagnosis with rapid molecular tests, free treatment with best quality drugs and regimens, financial and nutritional support to patients, online TB notification systems, mobile technology-based adherence monitoring system, interphase agencies for better private sector engagements, policy for transparent service purchase schemes, stronger community engagements, communication campaigns, regulatory systems to capture information on all those consuming anti-TB drugs, etc.
- To provide access to patients in difficult-to-reach areas, both socially and geographically.
- Policy have been in place now for using rapid molecular testing for TB diagnosis and universal drug resistance testing; now we have GenXpert tests available in every district.
- Recently validation and field feasibility tests of a "Make in India" rapid molecular test—"Trunat" has been completed.
- Daily fixed dose course (FDC) regimen for drug-sensitive TB has been now used in India with mobile-based adherence monitoring system (99-DOTS). For DR-TB patients, bedaquiline have been introduced and shorter MDR-TB regimen will be used for treatment.
- Patient support such as nutritional support and financial enablers are ready to be rolled out through JAN scheme [Jan Dhan Yojana (bank account to citizen), Aadhar (unique identity card), Nikshay (electronic TB notification system) linked, direct beneficiary transfer of financial incentives or nutritional support to TB patients]. 20% of NSP budget has been earmarked for financial and nutritional support to TB patients and families.
- Health system strengthening is one of the top priorities; in the NSP we have included a section called "Build". For strengthening TB program management, we have now an efficient, transparent public finance management system (PFMS). An effective TB

surveillance system is being developed in the country and, in 2 years, we expect to have a state of-the-art TB surveillance system in place to better understand and react to local TB epidemic.
- In India, a series of scientific ventures, including development of newer vaccines, newer molecular diagnostics, and treatment regimens are underway.

STRUCTURE OF RNTCP

The RNTCP works at five levels: national level, state level, district level, subdistrict level, and peripheral health institution level.

National Level

At the central level, the RNTCP is managed by the Central TB Division (CTD) under Ministry of Health and Family Welfare (MoHFW). Joint Secretary of Health from the administrative arm of the MoHFW and a national program manager—Deputy Director General-TB (DDG-TB), is in-charge of RNTCP.[2,3] The CTD is assisted by six national level institutes, namely the National Tuberculosis Institute (NTI) in Bengaluru, the National Institute for Research in Tuberculosis (NIRT) in Chennai, the National Institute of TB and Respiratory Diseases (NITRD) in New Delhi, National Japanese Leprosy Mission for Asia (JALMA), Institute of Leprosy and other Mycobacterial Diseases in Agra, Bhopal Memorial Hospital and Research Centre (BMHRC) in Bhopal, and Regional Medical Research Centre (RMRC) in Bhubaneswar.

State Level

At the state level, the state TB officer (STO) does the planning, training, supervising, and monitoring of the program in their respective states. The STO, based at the state TB cell, is answerable to their respective state governments, whilst implementing the technical policies and guidelines issued by the CTD. The state TB cells (STC) have been provided with equipment, infrastructure, and RNTCP contractual staff to carry out its functions. The State TB Training and Demonstration Centre (STDC) has three units: A training unit, supervision, and monitoring unit and an intermediate reference laboratory (IRL). There is state drug store (SDS) for the effective management of anti-TB drug logistics. One SDS per 50 million populations is established in all larger states.

District Level

The District TB Centre (DTC) is the nodal point for all TB control activities in the district. In RNTCP, the primary role of the DTC has shifted from clinical to managerial functions. The district TB officer (DTO) at the DTC has the overall responsibility of management of RNTCP at the district level as per the program guidelines and the guidance of the District Health Society.

Subdistrict Level (Tuberculosis Unit Level)

The tuberculosis unit consists of a designated Medical Officer-Tuberculosis Control (MO-TC) who does RNTCP work in addition to other responsibilities. There are two full-time RNTCP contractual supervisory staff exclusively for TB work: A Senior TB Treatment Supervisor (STS) and a Senior TB Laboratory Supervisor (STLS). These tuberculosis units cover a population of approximately 200,000–250,000.

There is one RNTCP designated microscopy center (DMC) for every 100,000 population under a TB unit (50,000 in tribal, desert, remote, and hilly regions). DMCs are also established in medical colleges, corporate hospitals, Employees State Insurance Corporation hospitals and railway health facilities, NGOs, private hospitals, etc., depending upon the requirement.

Peripheral Health Institutions

For the purpose of RNTCP, a peripheral health institution (PHI) is a health facility which is manned by at least a medical officer.

CASE DEFINITIONS

The RNTCP has developed clear definitions for pulmonary TB cases that allow clinicians to categorize patients in terms of their diagnostic status and outcomes of treatment.

Many TB patients do not have their diagnosis confirmed by a positive microbiological test either due to the limitations of the diagnostic tests currently available, or lack of access to a microbiological test. These patients are often treated based on the clinician's suspicion alone (empirical treatment).

Case Definitions

- Microbiologically confirmed TB case refers to a presumptive TB patient with biological specimen positive for acid fast bacilli, or positive for *Mycobacterium tuberculosis* on culture, or positive for TB through quality assured rapid diagnosis molecular test.
- Clinically diagnosed TB case refers to presumptive TB patient who is microbiologically confirmed, he has been diagnosed with active TB by a clinician on the basis of X-ray abnormalities. Histopathology or clinical signs with the design to treat the patient with full course of anti-TB treatment.

In children, clinically diagnosed TB case is diagnosed based on the presence of abnormalities consistent with TB radiography a history of exposure to an infectious case, evidence of TB infection [Positive tuberculin skin test (TST)] and clinical findings suggestive of TB in children in event of negative or unavailable microbiological result.

Microbiologically confirmed or clinically diagnosed case of TB are also classified according to:
- Anatomical site of disease
- History of previous treatment.

Classification based on anatomical site of disease:
- Pulmonary tuberculosis (PTB) refers to any microbiologically confirmed or clinically diagnosed case of TB involving the lungs parenchyma or tracheobronchial tree.
- Extrapulmonary tuberculosis (EPTB) refers to microbiologically confirmed or clinically diagnosed case of TB involving organ other than the lungs such as pleura, lymph nodes, intestine, genitor urinary tract, joint and bones, meninges of brain, etc.
- Miliary TB is classified such as PTB because there are lesions in the lungs. A patient with both PTB and EPTB should be classified as case of PTB.

Classification based on history of TB treatment:
- *New case*: A TB patient who has never had treatment for TB or has taken anti-TB drug for < 1 month is considered as new case.
- Previously treated patient has received 1 month or more of anti-TB drug in the past.

- *Recurrent TB case*: A TB patient previously declared as successfully treated, cured or treatment completed and subsequently found to be microbiologically confirmed TB case is recurrent TB case.
- *Treatment after loss to follow up*: A TB patient previously treated for TB for 1 month or more and was declared lost to follow-up in their most recent course of treatment and subsequently found microbiologically confirmed TB case.
- Other previously treated patients are those who have previously been treated for TB but whose outcome after their most recent course of treatment is unknown or undocumented.
- *Transferred in*: A TB patient who has received treatment in tuberculosis unit, after being registered for treatment in another TB unit is considered as case of transferred in.

Classification based on drug resistance:
- *Mono resistance (MR)*: A TB patient whose biological specimen is resistant to one first line anti-TB drug only.
- *Poly drug resistance (PDR)*: A TB patient whose specimen is resistant to more than one first line anti-TB drug, other than both isoniazid (INH) and rifampicin.
- *Multidrug resistance*: A TB whose biological specimen is resistant to both isoniazid and rifampicin with or without resistance to other first-line drug based on the result from a quality assured laboratory.
- *Extensive drug resistance (XDR)*: An MDR-TB case whose biological specimen is additionally resistance to a fluoroquinolone (ofloxacin, levofloxacin, or moxifloxacine) and a second line injectable anti-TB drug (kanamycin, amikacin, or capreomycin).

DEFINITION UNDER RNTCP

Working Case Definitions

Presumptive case: A patient with symptoms and signs of EPTB who needs investigation

Bacteriologically confirmed case: A patient with microbiological diagnosis of EPTB, based on positive microscopy, culture or a validated PCR (polymerase chain reaction)-based test.

Clinically diagnosed case: A patient with negative microbiological tests for TB (microscopy, culture and validated PCR-based tests), but with strong clinical suspicion and other evidence of EPTB, such as compatible imaging findings, histological findings, ancillary diagnostic tests or response to anti-TB treatment. A presumptive case started on antitubercular therapy (ATT) empirically, without microbiological testing, should also be considered a clinically diagnosed case (empirically treated). A clinically diagnosed case subsequently found to be bacteriologically positive (before or after starting treatment) should be reclassified as bacteriologically confirmed.

Non-EPTB case: A patient who has been investigated for EPTB and has been diagnosed with a different condition, with no microbiological evidence of EPTB found.

Presumptive relapse: A patient who was declared successfully treated and now presents again with symptoms and signs of any form of TB.

Bacteriologically confirmed relapse: A patient with presumptive relapse who has microbiological evidence of persisting *M. tuberculosis* infection on subsequent diagnostic sampling.

Clinically diagnosed relapse: A patient with presumptive relapse who does not have microbiological evidence of persisting *M. tuberculosis* infection on repeat diagnostic sampling.

A patient with presumptive relapse who is started on ATT empirically without repeat microbiological tests should also be considered a clinically diagnosed relapse (empirically treated). A clinically diagnosed relapse subsequently found to be bacteriologically positive (before or after starting treatment) should be reclassified as bacteriologically confirmed relapse.

Ancillary diagnostic tests refer to organ system-specific tests such as pleural fluid adenosine deaminase activity (ADA) in pleural TB, or cerebrospinal fluid (CSF) biochemistry and differential cell count in TB meningitis.

Working Outcome Definitions[1]

Successfully treated: A TB patient who has clinical and radiological evidence of resolution of active TB at the end of ATT. Some people have residual tissue damage that causes ongoing symptoms or radiological change (sequelae) despite resolution of TB infection.

Completed treatment: A TB patient who completed treatment without clinical evidence of failure but with no record to show complete resolution by radiological or bacteriological evidence of persisting infection by the last month of treatment because tests were not done.

Presumptive treatment failure: A patient who has no satisfactory clinical or imaging response to treatment after completing 3-6 months ATT.

Bacteriologically confirmed treatment failure: A patient with presumptive treatment failure who has microbiological evidence of persisting *M. tuberculosis* infection on repeat diagnostic sampling.

Clinically diagnosed treatment failure: A presumptive treatment failure case who does not have microbiological evidence of persisting *M. tuberculosis* infection on repeat diagnostic sampling and has no evidence of another disease process, but has strong clinical suspicion of treatment failure and other evidence of active TB, such as imaging findings.

SEQUELAE OF EXTRAPULMONARY TUBERCULOSIS

The difficulty in defining treatment end-points in EPTB is due to the development of sequelae as a result of the inflammation and subsequent fibrosis.[4] Patients with sequelae though may have complete microbiological cure, but continue to have symptoms. In EPTB at times, sequelae can mimic the signs and symptoms of active TB infection, and to declare the patient successfully treated difficult.

LABORATORY

Early accurate diagnosis of TB and enhancing case finding efficiency, identification of presumptive TB cases and avail the best available diagnostic tests are of paramount importance to interrupt the transmission of TB disease. RNTCP screens around 20 million TB symptomatic by microscopy and initiates around 1.5 million cases of TB on treatment annually since 2007-2008. Rapid molecular diagnostics and line probe assay and cartridge based-nucleic acid amplification test (CBNAAT) testing is available throughout the country. In 2016, 520,000 patients have been tested and 35,000 rifampicin resistant (RR)/MDR-TB patients are diagnosed using these tests. Second-line drug susceptibility testing (DST) using liquid culture systems are available in the entire country. RNTCP has a three-tier laboratory network system. The National Reference Laboratory (NRL), IRL, DMCs, and all the laboratories under RNTCP follow the quality assurance (QA) protocol for all technologies as per the WHO guidelines.

The program has a very well established QA mechanism which follows the WHO system of hierarchal control from the highest level of NRLs to state.

TREATMENT SERVICE

Strengthening of these patient-centered treatment services in RNTCP with enhanced capacity to rapidly accommodate new drugs and treatment modalities will be the cornerstone of the current NSP.

Patients are classified based on drug sensitive and drug-resistant patterns like mono, poly, multi, and extensive drug resistance. For drug-sensitive TB patients, thrice-weekly regimen being followed since program inception has been switched to daily regimen for treatment of all TB patients.

The principles of treatment for TB are:
- Compulsory screening of all patients for rifampicin-resistance and additional drugs as clinically decided.
- For drug-sensitive TB, administer daily fixed dose combinations of first-line anti-tuberculosis drugs including four-drug fixed-dose combinations (FDCs) in the intensive phase and three-drug FDCs in the continuation phase.
- All RR or MDR-TB patients are subjected to baseline kanamycin and levofloxacin.
- Rifampicin-resistant or MDR-TB patients without additional drug resistance are treated with standard short course treatment regimen for MDR-TB. and, mixed patterns of resistance, standard MDR-TB regimens were modified.
- Essential optimized regimen for patients diagnosed with drug resistance other than MDR- and XDR-TB.
- Maximize adherence through innovative patient support strategies and real time monitoring.

As part of new drug and treatment services introduction, the program plans to introduce shorter MDR-TB regimen as per WHO treatment guidelines. With extended DST for second-line drugs being available upfront, the NSP 2017–2025 also envisages countrywide scale up of new drugs like bedaquiline (being currently provided in six sites across the country) and delamanid.

PROGRAMMATIC MANAGEMENT OF DRUG-RESISTANT TUBERCULOSIS

The World Health Organization's Global TB Report 2015 estimates approximately 71,000 cases of MDR-TB that emerge annually from the notified cases of pulmonary TB in India. Based on subnational drug resistance surveys carried out in three states of India, ~3% among new TB cases and 12–17% among previously-treated TB cases have MDR-TB.

Strategies for controlling DR-TB include: (i) Sustained high-quality DOTS implementation, daily regimen in high-risk groups and patient-friendly treatment to improve treatment adherence; (ii) implementing airborne infection control (AIC) measures; cut down diagnostic delays with rapid diagnostics, offer universal DST and prompt appropriate decentralized treatment; (iii) strengthening procurement, supply chain: Strengthen the procurement, supply and availability of second-line anti-TB drugs in India; (iv) nutritional assessment and supplementation: Linkages with public distribution systems, Panchayati Raj institutions, corporate social responsibility, etc.; and (v) improving adherence through counseling support: One DR-TB counselor per DR-TB center and district each for both institutional and home-based counseling.

The key features from programmatic management of DR-TB (PMDT) guidelines are described here.

Diagnosis of Multidrug or Extensively Drug-resistant TB

Decentralized diagnosis with with specimen transported to laboratory in cold chain. Rapid molecular DST [CBNAAT or line probe assay (LPA)] is the first choice of DST. All failures of first-line regimen, contacts of known MDR-TB case, all retreatment cases at diagnosis, any patient with smear positive follow up results, and all TB-HIV cases are offered DST.

Apart from these, presumptive TB cases among people living with HIV/AIDS (PLHA) are prioritized for early diagnosis of TB using CBNAAT and the resulting DR-TB cases detected are also considered for treatment under PMDT. Baseline second-line drug in confirmed MDR-TB cases with a fluoroquinolone and second-line injectables. The patients diagnosed with ofloxacin/kanamycin (Ofx/Km) resistance are treated with modified MDR-TB regimen whereas the Ofx/Km resistance among nonresponders and failures of MDR-TB regimen are treated with XDR-TB regimen.

Treatment of Multidrug or Extensively Drug-resistant Tuberculosis

Treatment is based on DR or DST results. Initial hospitalization is done at DR-TB center followed by ambulatory care. A standardized treatment regimen is used for MDR-TB—daily DOT that consists of 6–9 months of kanamycin; levofloxacin; cycloserine; ethionamide; pyrazinamide; ethambutol or 18 months of levofloxacin; cycloserine; ethionamide; ethambutol. Para-aminosalicylic acid (PAS) is used as a substitute drug in case of intolerance.

Standardized treatment regimen for XDR-TB—daily DOT, consisting of 6–12 months of capreomycin; PAS; moxifloxacin; high-dose isoniazid; clofazimine; linezolid; amoxycillin-clavulanic acid or 18 months of PAS, moxifloxacin, high-dose isoniazid, clofazimine; linezolid; amoxycillin-clavulanic acid. Clarithromycin and thiacetazone are used as a substitute drug in case of intolerance.

TUBERCULOSIS–HUMAN IMMUNODEFICIENCY VIRUS COLLABORATIVE ACTIVITIES

Tuberculosis is commonest opportunistic infection in HIV-infected individuals and HIV-infection is an important risk factor for acquiring TB infection and its progression to active TB. About 120,000 HIV-associated TB patients are emerging annually in India and accounts for about 10% of the global burden of HIV-associated TB. The mortality in among TB/HIV coinfected patients is 38,000 people every year.

The interventions to reduce the burden of TB among PLHA include the early provision of antiretroviral therapy (ART) for people living with HIV in line with WHO guidelines and the three I's for HIV/TB—intensified TB case finding followed by high quality ATT, isoniazid preventive therapy (IPT), and infection control for TB.

The National Framework for Joint TB-HIV Collaborative Activities was developed in 2007 and has been updated based on experiential learning and scientific evidence. Currently, the TB/HIV package is being implemented nationwide by both the programs.

PROGRESS SO FAR

In 2014, 74% TB patients knew their HIV status and 44,067 were diagnosed as HIV positive. The 93% HIV-TB patients were provided co-trimoxazole preventive therapy (CPT) and 91% coinfected patients are put on ART.

The 4% additional TB cases were diagnosed with intensified TB case finding activities at HIV care settings.

The success rate among the HIV-TB coinfected patients for patients registered in 2013 was 76% with high death rate 13% and default rate was 6%.

TUBERCULOSIS AND NONCOMMUNICABLE COMORBIDITIES (TOBACCO, DIABETES)

The increasing co-occurrence of TB with tobacco consumption and diabetes mellitus (DM) is well evident. Smoking is three times more prevalent in TB patients and is strongly associated with increased rates of TB infection. Similarly, the prevalence of DM is as high as 13% and the prevalence even goes higher in MDR-TB cases. Patients with TB may have lung damage that is aggravated by continued tobacco use.

Feasibility of including tobacco cessation activities with RNTCP, a TB tobacco pilot project was conducted in Gujarat by Government of India in 2010. The pilot projects done by the TB-DM collaborative group has demonstrated at eight tertiary care centers that missed opportunities can be addressed through developing routine screening system in RNTCP with no additional cost to program.

CHILDHOOD TUBERCULOSIS

As per the Global Report on TB 2014, there were an estimated 550,000 TB cases among children (under 15 years of age) and 80,000 TB deaths (among HIV-negative children) in 2013 (6% and 8% of the global totals, respectively). It is one of the top 10 causes of childhood mortality.

Revised National TB Control Programme in association with Indian Academy of Pediatrics (IAP) has revised the pediatric TB guideline in 2012. It laid down specific algorithm diagnosis of TB among children. The treatment strategy comprises two key components. First, as in adults, children with TB are treated with standard SCC, given under direct observation and the disease status is monitored during the course of treatment. Second, patient wise boxes designed according to weight bands for complete course of anti-TB drugs.

In 2014, 72,307 new TB cases were notified accounting for 6% of all cases. This is in the range of the expected incidence by WHO report. The contact screening is one of the ways for intensified case finding activity which RNTCP has implemented since its inception.

The National Technical Working Group on pediatric TB has been constituted to examine the policy and practices and provides suggestions to CTD for improving situation of childhood TB.

To accelerate access to quality TB diagnosis for pediatric, RNTCP has initiated a project in four major cities in India': RNTCP United States Agency for International Development (USAID) Foundation for Innovative New Diagnostics (FIND) Pediatric TB Xpert Project.

PUBLIC–PRIVATE MIX DOTS IN RNTCP

In India, the private sector is the first point of care in many episodes of ill health. While most TB cases are ultimately treated by the RNTCP, most patients by then have already approached the private sector for TB diagnosis and treatment.

After experiences of implementing models of private sector collaboration, CTD published guidelines for the participation of the NGOs (in 2001) and private practitioners (in 2002). Currently, 24 partnership options for involvement of NGOs, corporates, private practitioners and research institutions are incorporated under the National Guidelines for Partnership.

Indian Medical Association has been engaged with the program through Global Fund to Fight AIDS, Tuberculosis and Malaria (GFATM) supported project in 16 states and union territories. Similarly, civil society organization, CBCI-CARD (The Catholic Bishops' Conference of India-Coalition for AIDS and Related Diseases) is working under GFATM project of RNTCP, to improve access to the diagnostic and treatment services provided by the RNTCP within the Catholic Church Healthcare Facilities (CHFs).

In addition, partners like UNION, World Vision, and FIND also support the program. RNTCP has partnered with more than 350 medical colleges in India and, in 2014, they have contributed in a major way in finding more TB cases, especially smear negative and EPTB cases.

ADVOCACY COMMUNICATION AND SOCIAL MOBILIZATION

Advocacy communication and social mobilization (ACSM) is an inbuilt component of RNTCP and is recognized as an important element.

Information, education and communication (IEC) materials are developed at the national level and shared with states for use—"as it is" or post modification to suit local requirements. Several of these materials including television spots, radio jingles and posters are available in nearly 13 regional languages. Advocacy communication and social mobilization module is incorporated in all health workers training on basic DOTS.

TUBERCULOSIS-PATIENT SUPPORT SYSTEMS IN INDIA

In addition to better diagnostic tool and treatment regimens, other patient supportive initiatives including better nutrition, counseling and financial support are equally essential. WHO's "End TB strategy" has this important target of "no affected family face catastrophic costs due to TB".

However, the free diagnosis and treatment is only accessible to those patients seeking care under RNTCP. Large number of patients seeking care in private sector has to bear substantial cost for TB care. Though large part of cost of treatment is borne by the program, patients still have to bear expenditures such as cost for travel to the facilities, loss of wages due to sickness, etc. The support activities are implemented through departments such as social welfare department, public distribution system, NGOs, CSR funding, etc.

PREVENTION

Airborne Infection Control

Acute respiratory infections (ARIs) are the leading cause of morbidity and mortality affecting the youngest and oldest people in low- and middle-income nations. These infections, typically caused by viruses or mixed viral–bacterial infections, can be contagious and spread rapidly. Although knowledge of transmission modes is ever-evolving, current evidence indicates that the primary mode of transmission of most acute respiratory diseases is through droplets, but transmission through contact (including hand contamination followed by self-inoculation) or infectious respiratory aerosols at short range can also happen for some pathogens in particular circumstances.

Contact Tracing

In RNTCP, contact screening has been a clinical function and the end result expected is that most TB patients will have their contacts screened, with secondary cases detected and treated.

Contact investigation:
- All close contacts, especially household contacts by X-rays
- In case of pediatric TB patients, reverse contact tracing for active TB case in the household of the child.

Use of chest X-rays upfront for screening of contacts will be prioritized during the NSP period. Setting specific screening approaches (for example in prisons, urban slums, etc.) according to the RNTCP technical and operational guidelines (TOG) will be undertaken.

All close contacts of DR-TB cases will be identified through contact tracing and evaluated for active TB disease as per RNTCP guidelines. If the contact is found to be suffering from pulmonary TB disease irrespective of the smear results, he will be identified as "presumptive MDR-TB".

Preventive Therapy or Latent Tuberculosis Infection Treatment

Tuberculosis infection is the seedbed for developing TB disease and continued transmission. The lifetime risk of reactivation of latent tuberculosis infection (LTBI) in healthy HIV-uninfected individuals is 10%, with 5% developing TB disease during the first 2–5 years after infection. The risk of reactivation is greatly increased in the context of immunosuppression, primarily due to HIV infection. Child contacts living in TB-affected households are particularly vulnerable populations for progression to TB and severe disease forms such as disseminated and meningeal TB. WHO has included scaling up TB preventive therapy for persons at high risk of developing TB in its End TB strategy and increasing coverage of contact investigations and TB preventive therapy for people living with HIV (PLHIV) and child contacts are important strategies. Scaling up TB preventive therapy is therefore important to meet the goals of ending TB in India.

India, with one-fourth of the global burden of TB, has 40% of the population infected with M. tuberculosis. Treating 40% of the population for LTBI based on TST positivity or interferon-gamma release assay is neither rational nor practicable, thus emphasizing the need for a focused approach. The selection of the risk group that will be prioritized for screening, investigation to rule out TB and treatment is as follows:
- People living with HIV
- Child PTB contacts
- Patients with silicosis
- All patients where clinically indicated (high risk), e.g., points in immunosuppressants
- High-risk adult contacts.

Isoniazid Preventive Therapy

Children <6 years of age, who are close contacts of a TB patient, will be evaluated for active TB by a medical officer/pediatrician. After excluding active TB, he/she will be given INH preventive therapy irrespective of their Bacillus Calmette-Guérin (BCG) vaccine or nutritional status. The dose of INH for preventive therapy is 10 mg/kg body weight daily for 6 months be collected on monthly basis. INH preventive therapy:
- For all HIV infected children with known exposure to an infectious TB case or are TST positive (≥5 mm induration) but have no active TB disease.
- All TST-positive children receiving immunosuppressive therapy (e.g., children with nephrotic syndrome, acute leukemia, etc.).

REFERENCES

1. Ministry of Health and Family Welfare. (2017). National Strategic Plan for Tuberculosis Elimination 2017-2025. Revised National Tuberculosis Control Programme. [online] Available from https://tbcindia.gov.in/WriteReadData/NSP%20Draft%2020.02.2017%201.pdf. [Last accessed January, 2020].
2. MGMIS Sevagram. (2018). National Strategic Plan (NSP) for Tuberculosis Step Towards ending TB by 2025. [online] Available from http://www.jmgims.co.in/article.asp?issn=0971-9903;year=2019;volume=24;issue=1;spage=17;epage=18;aulast=Khaparde. [Last accessed January, 2020].
3. Revised National Tuberculosis Control Programme Technical and Operational Guideline 2016, Directorate General of Health Services, MOHFW, New Delhi.
4. Sharma SK, Ryan H, Khaparde S, Sachdeva KS, Singh AD, Mohan A, et al. Index TB: Guidelines for extra pulmonary tuberculosis in India. 2017;145(4):448-63.

CHAPTER 2

Excerpts from Guidelines on Management of Drug-resistant Tuberculosis

Sujata Patwardhan, Narendra Sutar

"Taken from the Revised National Tuberculosis Control Programme, Central TB Division, Directorate General of Health Services, Ministry of Health and Family Welfare, Nirman Bhavan, New Delhi."

These national guidelines are available on the internet; however, they pertain to pulmonary tuberculosis (TB).[1-5]

Not every consultant or student have time to access to this guidelines and hence certain sections relevant to genitourinary TB (GUTB) and important parts of these guidelines are included in this chapter to help in understanding of our national program and be a part of it by following the guidelines.

The salient topics covered are:
1. Definitions and classification of drug-resistant TB (DR-TB) patients
2. State-level structure and responsibilities
3. Methods for drug-susceptibility testing (DST)
4. Choice of diagnostic technology
5. Specimen collection and transportation to culture and drug-susceptibility testing (C-DST) laboratories
6. Integrated DR-TB diagnostic algorithm
7. Treatment of drug-resistant TB
8. Newer anti-TB drugs
9. Regulatory approvals for bedaquiline in India
10. Integrated DR-TB algorithm
11. Management of DR-TB in extrapulmonary TB patients
12. Management of contacts of DR-TB
13. RNTCP laboratory register for culture, CBNAAT, and DST
14. RNTCP PMDT referral for treatment form
15. NIKSHAY
16. Infection control measures
17. References for further reading

DEFINITIONS AND CLASSIFICATION OF DRUG-RESISTANT TUBERCULOSIS PATIENTS

The following are the definitions and classification for DR-TB patients:

Presumptive DR-TB:

It refers to the following patients in order of their risk:
- TB patients found positive on any follow-up sputum smear examination during treatment with first-line drugs including treatment failures.
- Pediatric TB nonresponders
- TB patients who are contacts of DR-TB
- Previously treated TB patients
- New TB patients with HIV co-infection
- All notified new TB patients

A patient is confirmed to have DR-TB only when the results are from a Revised National Tuberculosis Control Programme (RNTCP) quality-assured C-DST laboratory and by a RNTCP-endorsed testing method. Such patients are classified according to the following definitions:

- *Mono-resistant TB* (MR-TB): A TB patient, whose biological specimen is resistant to one first line anti-TB drug only.
- *Poly-drug resistant TB* (PDR-TB): A TB patient, whose biological specimen is resistant to more than one first-line anti-TB drug, other than both H and R.

Although new TB patients from above-mentioned categories are at the lower risk of drug resistance, testing them further for presence of drug resistance at the time of diagnosis is a necessary standard of care.

- *Rifampicin resistance* (RR): A TB patient, whose biological specimen is resistant to R, detected using phenotypic or genotypic methods, with or without resistance to other anti-TB drugs. It includes any resistance to R, in the form of MR, poly-resistance, MDR, or XDR.
- *Multidrug resistance* (MDR): A TB patient, whose biological specimen is resistant to both H and R with or without resistance to other first-line anti-TB drugs. MDR-TB patients may also have additional resistance to any/all FQ OR any/all second-line injectable (SLI) anti-TB drugs.
- *Extensive drug resistance* (XDR): A MDR-TB patient whose biological specimen is additionally resistant to at least a FQ (Ofx, Lfx, Mfx) and a SLI anti-TB drug (Km, Am, and Cm).

It is to be noted that R resistance is quite rare without H resistance. Majority of DST results with R resistance will also be H resistant, i.e., MDR-TB. This has been substantiated in the National Drug Resistance Survey (2014–16).[6] Therefore, RNTCP has taken the programmatic decision that patients, who have any R resistance, should be managed as if they are an MDR-TB patient and this is in line with the World Health Organization (WHO) global guidelines for the programmatic management of drug-resistant TB (PMDT).

STATE-LEVEL STRUCTURE AND RESPONSIBILITIES

The National Expert Technical Working Group has developed national policies, and technical and operational guidelines. The state level is where the majority of planning activities, implementation, and monitoring occur. The State PMDT Committee is responsible for developing the plan of action for implementation, expansion, maintenance, and supervision, monitoring and quality enhancement of PMDT services in the respective state.

Drug-resistant Tuberculosis Center

Treatment of DR-TB is not completely based on centralized and institutionalized care for the entire duration. In fact, clinical care needs the presence of a clinical and patient support expert resource center. This is the DRTBC which is a 20–30-bedded tertiary care facility established to serve a population of approximately 10 million, with an airborne infection.

Overall PMDT structures and roles are:
- Diagnose rifampicin-resistant patients at district level
- Receive diagnostic/follow-up specimens
- Provide rapid results to district field and DR-TB center
- Maintain records and NIKSHAY
- Quality assurance of results
- Maintain ward and airborne infection control (AIC) measures
- Pretreatment evaluation
- Start MDR/XDR-TB treatment
- Consult for complications
- Clinical expert resource
- Maintain records and NIKSHAY
- Identify suspects and refer specimens
- Coordinate for test results
- Refer patients to N/DDR-TBC (nodal/district DR-TB center)
- Coordinate care and drug flow from district drug store to field level
- Maintain records, NIKSHAY, monitor, and supervise
- Prepare and ship drug boxes to district level
- Manage supply chain for diagnostics and drugs
- Maintain records, NIKSHAY, and DVDMS (Drug vaccine distribution management system)
- Initiate patient on standard DRTB regimen (MDR/RR-TB, H mono-/poly-DR-TB patients)
- Manage adverse drug reaction (ADR)
- Maintain records and NIKSHAY
- Identify presumptive case and refer specimens
- Support, supervise, and manage DR-TB patients
- Communicate results to patients
- Manage minor adverse effects
- Refer patient for the treatment initiation
- Collect and refer follow-up specimens.

METHODS FOR DRUG SUSCEPTIBILITY TESTING

Presently, drug resistance detection using the following technologies is available for diagnosis of DR-TB through rapid molecular diagnostic testing:

Line probe assay (LPA) for detection of *Mycobacterium tuberculosis* (MTB) complex and resistance to first-line drugs R, H and second-line drugs class FQ and class SLI drugs[7,8] and cartridge-based nucleic acid amplification test (CBNAAT) Xpert MTB/rifampicin testing using the GeneXpert platform for now.[8]

Growth-based phenotypic drug susceptibility testing: Culture, though a highly sensitive and specific method for TB diagnosis, requires 2–8 weeks to yield results and hence does not help in early detection. However, culture will be used for long-term follow-up of patients on DR-TB treatment and help detect early recurrence in both drug-sensitive and DR-TB. The growth-based phenotypic culture methods include automated liquid culture (LC) systems, e.g., BACTEC MGIT 960, BacT/Alert or VersaTREK, and solid [Löwenstein–Jensen (LJ)] media.

Rapid molecular drug resistance testing: LPA provides rapid diagnosis of R and H resistance as well as resistance to class FQ and class SLI drugs. LPA can yield results in 72 hours.

Nucleic acid amplification test (NAAT) provides accurate and rapid diagnosis of TB by detecting MTB and R resistance conferring mutations.[8] The test can be performed on both respiratory and nonrespiratory specimens and yield results in 2 hours. Presently, under RNTCP, its use is recommended for diagnosis of DR-TB in presumptive DR-TB patients and TB in children, extrapulmonary TB (EPTB) and in key population such as people living with HIV (PLHIV), socially and clinically vulnerable groups and for active case finding efforts.

Drug resistance status is determined by either of the following methods:
- *Drug resistance tests (DRTs) using molecular methods*: This can be performed on sputum specimen (direct) or on culture isolates (indirect) for diagnostic purpose. The methods are PCR-based and cannot be used for determining response to treatment. The tests that belong to this group include:
  - CBNAAT: It can be performed on smear-positive, smear-negative and EP specimens. The test detects TB and resistance to R LPA is performed on smear-positive specimen. The test detects TB and resistance to R and H [first-line LPA (FL-LPA)] as well as class FQ and class SLI [second-line LPA (SL-LPA)].
- *Drug susceptibility test*: These are growth based tests and can be performed on LJ culture isolates or in LC system mycobacteria growth indicator tube (MGIT) for both pulmonary and EP specimen. Most commonly used method for testing is the economic variant of the proportion sensitivity. MGIT is preferred method for DST and both first- and second-line anti-TB drugs can be tested. Following drugs can be tested for susceptibility by LC:
  - First-line drugs: R, H, Z*
  - Second-line drugs: Lfx, Mfx, Km, Cm, Am -
  - Other drugs: Lzd, Cfz*, Bdq*, Dlm*, etc.

*When standardized, the WHO endorsed and approved for use in program.

CHOICE OF DIAGNOSTIC TECHNOLOGY

The program has substantially scaled up the laboratory capacity of various C-DST laboratories. The choice of technology to be used for diagnosis of DR-TB has been determined as per recommendations of the National Laboratory Committee. The choice of technologies is given in the following text.

Drug Resistance Diagnostic Technology Choice

Following are the choices for drug resistance diagnostic technology:
- *First*: CBNAAT/LPA
- *Second*: LC isolation and LPA DST
- *Third*: LC isolation and liquid DST

All the follow-up cultures will be done through the LC. If the state is facing challenges, with respect to follow-up culture by LC, this may be communicated to the Central TB Division for facilitation.

Specimen Collection and Transportation to C-DST Laboratories

Obtaining good quality specimens of adequate volume is critical to ensuring correct diagnosis. Though the guidelines are specifically mentioned only sputum, the same are applicable to a collected specimen. The Laboratory technician needs to explain the process of collecting "a good-quality sputum specimen" while adhering to AIC measures. The program recommends collection of sputa one spot and one morning, OR two spot specimens collected within a gap of at least 1 hour (if the patient is coming from a long distance OR she/he is unlikely to return to give the second specimen). Ideally, a sputum specimen should have a volume of 2–5 mL and preferably be mucopurulent. Care should be taken to ensure that specimens sent for molecular testing are not heavily blood stained or contaminated. It is advisable to let the hemoptysis subside before collecting the specimen. The patient must be advised to collect the specimen in a sterile container (50-mL conical tube) after thorough rinsing of the mouth with clean water. Specimens should be transported to the laboratory as soon as possible after collection. In case of leakage or spillage of specimen during transportation leading to nontesting of specimen, special care should be taken to ensure recollection of specimen.

As per the diagnostic algorithm, two fresh specimens need to be collected at designated collection centers [designated microscopy center (DMC) or peripheral health institute (PHI) level] by trained laboratory technician (LT) and transported in a cool chain on the same day to the nearest CBNAAT laboratory for all eligible patients. At the CBNAAT site, the test is performed. For all results reported as TB [rifampicin-susceptible (RS) and RR], the second specimen needs to be repacked by the CBNAAT LT and transported to the RNTCP C-DST laboratory on the same day in cool chain. The request form (RNTCP request form for examination of biological specimen for TB) updated with the CBNAAT result should be sent along with the transported specimen. Simultaneously, the result of CBNAAT test is to be communicated to the patient and provider. At the C-DST laboratory, SL-LPA is performed for RR-TB and FL-LPA for RS-TB. All specimens need to be delivered to the RNTCP C-DST laboratory within 48–72 hours of collection. Ideally, an agency (courier/speed post) should be identified for this purpose by the concerned district TB officer (DTO). NGOs may be engaged as per partnership guidelines for specimen transportation in cool chain. If none is available, transporter need to be identified from the health system/community to transport the specimen in biosafe conditions with appropriate enablers. Models for packaging specimens are given in **Figure 2.1**. The following points are critical for the collection of fresh sputum specimens at designated collection points:
- 50-mL conical bottom tubes (made of polypropylene material) and the three-layer packing materials such as thermocol box, ice gel pack (pre-freezed at −20°C for 48 hours), request form for examination of biological specimen for TB, polythene bags, tissue paper roll as absorbent, parafilm tapes, brown tape for packaging box,

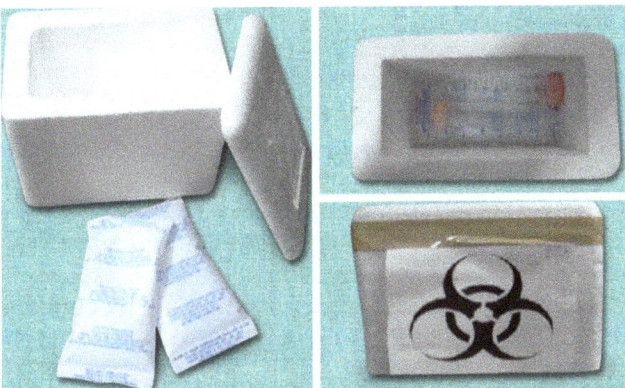

FIG. 1: Technical specifications of transport box for sputum specimen transportation in cool chain.

permanent marker pen, labels, BIOHAZARD sticker, scissors, and spirit swab should be supplied to the DMCs for collection of sputum through the DTO.
- About 50-mL conical tubes should carry a label indicating the date of collection of the specimens along with patient's details such as name, date of specimen collection, name of DMC/District Tuberculosis Center (DTC), Lab. No:- XYZ, and specimen A or B.
- Laboratory technician at DMCs should be trained to carefully to pack the sputum specimens in the cool box to avoid spillage of the specimens.
- Laboratory technician of DMC issuing the conical tubes to the patients should give clear instructions to the patients on correct technique of collection of the sputum. Also the date of issue of the conical tubes to the patient should be recorded.
- Laboratory technician of DMC should ensure that the request form for examination of biological specimen for TB is packed in a separate plastic zip pouch and placed in the cool box before sealing the lid of the box. Also, the BIOHAZARD symbol should be pasted on the external side of the cool box along with the label indicating the postal address of the C-DST laboratory assigned.
- Laboratory technician of DMC should promptly inform the specimen transport agency such as a courier/speed post service to collect and transport the specimens.
- As per national guidelines on biomedical waste management the containers used for transporting sputum specimens to the C-DST laboratory should be labeled with a "BIOHAZARD" sticker.

INTEGRATED DR-TB DIAGNOSTIC ALGORITHM

The vision of the program is to offer DST to TB patients at the earliest time in their diagnostic process. The integrated diagnostic algorithm starts with two groups of patients who are either presumptive TB or diagnosed TB. The main objective of this algorithm is to segregate people based on risk assessment for DR-TB and offer DST-guided treatment based on drug-resistance status at least for R resistance at the time of diagnosis of TB, i.e., Universal DST. The subsequent time points when DST is offered if any of the following events occur during the course of a TB treatment schedule:

- Bacteriologically positive after intensive phase of a course of TB/DR-TB treatment
- Failure to respond to treatment as per RNTCP definitions
- Recurrence of TB diagnosed after a course of TB treatment
- For patients who are retrieved after lost to follow-up
- For patients found to be HIV positive before or anytime during the course of TB treatment
- Any other reason as per treating physicians' advice.

Two diagnostic specimens would be collected from the patients one early morning and one spot specimen wherever possible, but if there is a likelihood of the patient not returning for the second collection or traveling from long distance then two spot specimens may be collected with a gap of at least 1 hour. The DR-TB diagnostic algorithm is as given in **Flowchart 2.1**.

Persons presumed to have TB are:
- From this group those belonging to the pediatric age group
- PLHIV
- EP group or with a smear-negative chest X-ray suggestive of TB will be offered CBNAAT test.

By virtue of using CBNAAT as the TB diagnostic test, the R status is also available simultaneously along with TB detection.

The integrated DR-TB diagnostic algorithm 2020 guidelines has been shown in **Flowchart 2.2**.

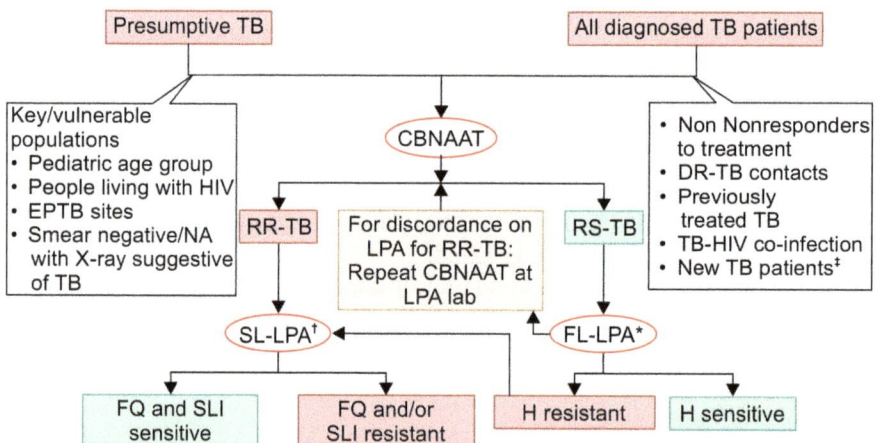

* Offer molecular testing for H mono/poly resistance to TB patients prioritized by risk as per the available lab capacity
† LC DST (Mfx 2.0, Km, Cm, Lzd) will be done only for patients with any resistance on baseline Sl-LPA. DST to Z, Cfz, BDQ and DLM would be considered for policy in future, whenever available, standardized and WHO endorsed.
‡ States to advance in phased manner as per PMDT Scale up plan for universal DST based on lab capacity and policy on use of diagnostics.

(CBNAAT: cartridge-based nucleic acid amplification test; DR-TB: drug-resistant TB; DST: drug-susceptibility testing; EPTB: extrapulmonary TB; FL-LPA: first-line line probe assay; FQ: fluoroquinolone; LC: liquid culture; NA: not available; PMDT: programmatic management of drug-resistant TB; RR-TB: rifampicin-resistant TB; RS: rifampicin-susceptible TB; SL-LPA: second-line line probe assay; SLI: second-line injectable; TB: tuberculosis)

FLOWCHART 2.1: Drug-resistant tuberculosis diagnostic algorithm guidelines 2019.

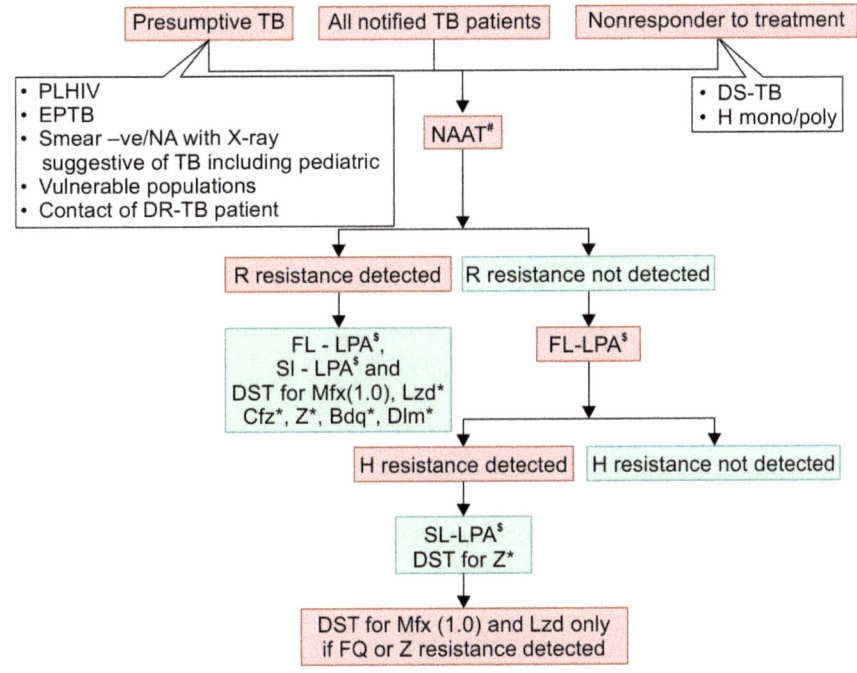

NAAT include CBNAAT and TruNAAT
* Whenever available
$ Culture isolated to be subjected to LPA for smear negative specimens

FLOWCHART 2.2: The integrated DR-TB diagnostic algorithm guidelines 2020.

TREATMENT OF DRUG-RESISTANT TUBERCULSOSIS

This section provides guidance on the treatment of all forms of DR-TB patients.

Classes of Anti-TB Drugs Recommended for Treatment of DR-TB Patients

The anti-TB drugs recommended for treatment of MDR/RR-TB patients are grouped based on efficacy, experience of use, and drug class and aligned with revised classification as per the WHO PMDT Guidelines 2016. The same is explained in **Table 2.1**.[9]

Newer Anti-TB Drugs

After almost five decades of discovery of rifampicin, the first new drug named bedaquiline (Bdq) with anti-TB effect was approved for treatment of MDR-TB by the US Food and Drug Administration (FDA) in late 2012.[10] This was followed by the approval of another new drug delamanid (DLM) by the stringent regulatory authority of various countries.[11] The drug development pipeline of new and repurposed drug has gained momentum in the recent past and more new molecules are expected to be approved in the future.

Bedaquiline is a new class of drug, diarylquinoline, that specifically targets mycobacterial ATP synthase, an enzyme essential for the supply of energy to MTB. Strong bactericidal and sterilizing activities against MTB have been shown in preclinical,

TABLE 2.1: Recommended anti-TB drugs for treat of MDR-/RR-TB patients.[3]

New grouping of drugs			
A. Fluoroquinolones		Levofloxacin	Lfx
		Moxifloxacin	Mfx
		Gatifloxacin	Gfx
B. Second-line injectable agents		Amikacin	Am
		Capreomycin	Cm
		Kanamycin	Km
		(Streptomycin)	(S)
C. Other second-line agents		Ethionamide/Prothionamide	Eto/Pto
		Cycloserine/Terizidone	Cs/Trd
		Linezolid	Lzd
		Clofazimine	Cfz
D. Add-on agents (not part of the core MDR-TB regimen)	D1	Pyrazinamide	Z
		Ethambutol	E
		High-dose isoniazid	H^h
	D2	Bedaquiline	Bdq
		Delamanid	Dim
	D3	p-aminosalicylic acid	PAS
		Imipenem-cilastatin	Ipm/Cls
		Meropenem	Mpm
		Amoxicillin-clavulanate	Amx-Clv
		(Thioacetazone)	(T)

(MDR-TB: multidrug-resistant tuberculosis; RR-TB: rifampicin-resistant TB)

laboratory, and animal experiments. The drug has a high volume of distribution, with extensive tissue distribution, highly bound to plasma proteins and is hepatically metabolized. The drug has an extended half-life, which means that it is still present in the plasma up to 5.5 months post stopping Bdq. The dosing schedule has been established after extensive pharmacokinetic/pharmacodynamic (PK/PD) studies in animals and humans and hence needs to be administered as per the manufacturer's advice. Bdq has shown significant benefits in improving the time to culture conversion in MDR-TB patients.[10]

Delamanid, as per an interim policy guidance document released by the WHO in 2014, may be added to a WHO-recommended regimen in adult patients with pulmonary MDR-TB.[11] The process for introduction of DLM under RNTCP is ongoing and guidance for the same will be released subsequently as an addendum to these guidelines.

Regulatory Approvals for Bedaquiline in India

On December 24, 2014, the Apex Committee under the Ministry of Health and Family Welfare, Government of India for supervising clinical trials on new chemical entities in the light of directions of the Supreme Court of India approved the use of Bdq (100 mg) in adults aged 18 years and above as part of a combination therapy of pulmonary TB due to MDR-TB.

Considering MDR-TB as a serious condition with high mortality and a disease of special relevance in the Indian health scenario, the committee recommended waiver of local clinical trials at this stage and approved Bdq with restriction that it shall be used under the RNTCP framework for conditional access through the PMDT program for treatment of MDR-TB patients only.

Criteria for Patients to Receive Bedaquiline

Inclusion criteria: The criterion for patients to receive Bdq as approved by the Apex Committee is—adults aged >18 years having pulmonary MDR-TB.

Additional requirements:
- Nonpregnant females or females not on hormonal birth control methods are eligible. They should be willing to continue practicing birth control methods throughout the treatment period or have been postmenopausal for past 2 years.
- Patients with controlled stable arrhythmia can be considered after obtaining cardiac consultation.

Exclusion criteria:
- Currently having uncontrolled cardiac arrhythmia that requires medication
- Having any of the following QT/QTc interval characteristics at screening—marked prolongation of QT/QTc interval, e.g., repeated demonstration of QTcF (Fredericia correction) interval >450 ms; and history of additional risk factors for Torsade de Pointes, e.g., heart failure, hypokalemia, family history of long QT syndrome.

Bedaquiline is provided along with a background regimen based on DST results. Certain conditions as listed below should be taken into consideration while choosing the drugs for the background regimen in patients who:
- Have evidence of chorioretinitis, optic neuritis, or uveitis at screening which precludes long-term Lzd therapy.
- Have the following laboratory abnormalities (DAIDS grading of adverse events):
    - Creatinine grade 2 or greater, i.e., >1.5 times the upper limit of normal (ULN);
    - Hemoglobin grade 4 (<6.5 g/dL)
    - Platelet count grade 3 or greater (≤49,999/mm^3);
    - Absolute neutrophils count grade 3 or greater (≤749/mm^3);
    - Aspartate aminotransferase (AST) grade 2 or greater (>2.5 times ULN)
    - Alanine aminotransferase (ALT) grade 2 or greater (>2.5 times ULN)
    - Total bilirubin grade 2 or greater (>1.6 times ULN)
    - Lipase grade 2 (with no signs or symptoms of pancreatitis) or greater (>1.5 times ULN).

Note: If results of the serum chemistry panel, hematology or urinalysis are outside the normal reference range (including above-listed parameters), the patient may still be considered if the physician judges abnormalities or deviations from normal to be not clinically significant or to be appropriate and reasonable. Hypokalemia, hypomagnesaemia, and hypocalcaemia should be corrected prior to a patient receiving Bdq.

Patients who are not found to be eligible for a Bdq-containing regimen would have DST results for the key first-line and second-line drugs and managed with DST-guided regimens.

Bedaquiline is indicated in adult MDR-TB patients not eligible for the newly WHO-recommended shorter regimen.[12]

These may include:
- MDR-/RR-TB patients with resistance to any/all FQ *OR* to any/all SLI
- XDR-TB patients

- Mixed pattern-resistant TB patients
- Treatment failures of MDR-TB + FQ/SLI resistance *OR* XDR-TB
- MDR-/RR-TB patients with extensive pulmonary lesions, advanced disease and others deemed at higher baseline risk for poor outcomes.[12]

Caution must be exercised that Bdq is not added to a failing regimen in any patient already on DR-TB treatment.

Integrated Drug-resistant Tuberculosis Algorithm

The integrated DR-TB algorithm (**Flowchart 2.1**) clearly indicates the management strategies to be followed right from the day the results of CBNAAT test are available. These management strategies are described in subsequent sections of this document. The program is improving laboratory capacity to offer DST for all TB patients (Universal DST). An integrated algorithm offers FL-LPA for the presumptive DR-TB found R sensitive on CBNAAT. The LPA will be primarily utilized to do DST for second-line drugs and to test FL-LPA to detect H mono-resistance as per the available laboratory capacity. The program would continue building capacity of the laboratories to eventually test all R-sensitive patients on LPA to detect H mono-resistance that would serve as a surrogate for poly-drug resistance. These patients would be managed as per the algorithm. Within the first 2–3 months, patients would receive the LC-DST results, reach their final classification, and treated with the appropriate regimen.

MANAGEMENT OF DR-TB IN EXTRAPULMONARY TB PATIENTS

Management of bacteriologically confirmed EP DR-TB patients will be considered by the program provided the diagnosis is made by an RNTCP C-DST laboratory. **Treatment regimen and schedule for EP DR-TB patients will remain the same as for pulmonary DR-TB**. Patients must be registered in the PMDT register and the treatment outcome of treatment completed will be considered.

Investigations and Pretreatment Evaluation

Patients would be sent to the DR-TBC for pretreatment evaluation and treatment initiation. EP DR-TB patients will undergo all those pretreatment investigations as done for pulmonary DR-TB patients as part of pretreatment evaluation prior to initiating regimen for DR-TB.

In addition, ultrasound of abdomen of the patient will also be done, if necessary, to rule out involvement of other organs and abdominal nodes. If required, additional imaging investigation will be done to rule out any other conditions.

Initiation of Treatment

After pretreatment evaluation, treatment for EP DR-TB should be initiated based on weight of the patient. Treatment regimen, weight band, and schedule for EP DR-TB patients will remain the same as for pulmonary DR-TB.

Monitoring Progress During Treatment and Follow-up

Post treatment monitoring and follow up recommended for MDR/RR-TB patients both pulmonary and extra pulmonary as well as for paediatric TB cases are based on classification as per the WHO PMDT guidelines 2016. The same is explained in **Table 2.2**.

Excerpts from Guidelines on Management of Drug-resistant Tuberculosis

TABLE 2.2: Follow-up schedule.

Type of cases	Follow-up schedule	Extension of treatment	Action on follow-up positive	Long-term follow-up
Drug-sensitive pulmonary TB (New and Previously treated TB)	• Microbiological: One specimen at the time of completion of the intensive phase of treatment • Weight: Monthly • Chest X-ray: If required • Physician evaluation: Whenever required	Extension of IP is not required	If the sputum smear is positive in follow-up at any time during treatment, DST should be done as per presumptive DR-TB case	After completion of treatment the patients should be followed up with clinical and/or sputum examination at the end of 6, 12, 18, and 24 months
Multidrug-resistant pulmonary TB (with or without additional drug resistance)	• Microbiological: One sputum specimen will be collected and examined by culture at least 30 days apart from the 3rd to 7th month of treatment (i.e., at the end of the months 3, 4, 5, 6, and 7) and at 3-monthly intervals from the 9th month onwards till the completion of treatment (i.e., at the end of the months 9, 12, 15, 18, 21, and 24). If any culture during CP or end of treatment is positive then it should be followed by monthly culture for 3 months • Weight: Monthly • Chest X-ray: At the end of IP, end of treatment and whenever clinically indicated • Physician evaluation including adverse drug reaction monitoring every month for 6 months, then every 3 months for 2 years	• In MDR-TB cases IP can be extended for maximum 3 months (maximum duration of IP: 9 months). • In all MDR-TB with additional drug resistant cases (including XDR-TB) patients, IP can be extended for maximum 6 months (maximum duration of IP: 12 months)	On follow-up, if sputum culture is found to be positive at 6 months or later, repeat DST for second-line drugs to decide on further course of action. DST to other additional second line drugs may also be done if laboratory facilities are available to guide treatment	

Continued

Continued

Type of cases	Follow-up schedule	Extension of treatment	Action on follow-up positive	Long-term follow-up
	• S. creatinine monthly for first 3 months then every 3 months during the injectable phase • Thyroid function test during pretreatment evaluation and whenever indicated • For additional drug resistance: ECG once a month in IP whenever moxifloxacin is used • Complete blood count with platelets count: Weekly in first month, then monthly to rule out bone marrow suppression and anemia as a side effect of Linezolid • Renal function test: Monthly creatinine and addition on monthly serum electrolytes to the monthly creatinine during the period then injection capreomycin is being administered • Liver function tests: Monthly in IP and 3 monthly during CP • Chest X-ray: Every 6 months in XDR-TB patients			
Mono- /Poly- drug resistant Pulmonary TB	Microbiological: One sputum specimen is collected and examined with smear and culture at 2nd and 3rd months and then culture examination at 3 monthly intervals till completion of treatment	IP can be extended for maximum 3 months (maximum duration of IP: 6 months)	If the sputum/culture is positive in follow up at any time during treatment, DST should be done as per presumptive DR-TB case	After completion of treatment the patients should be followed up with clinical and/or sputum examination at the end of 6, 12, 18, and 24 months

Continued

Type of cases	Follow-up schedule	Extension of treatment	Action on follow-up positive	Long-term follow-up
Extrapulmonary TB	• Weight: Monthly • Chest X-ray: If required • Physician evaluation: Whenever required • In patients with extrapulmonary tuberculosis, the treatment response is best assessed clinically. The help of radiological and other relevant investigations may also be taken as above	• Extension of IP or and/or CP in DS-EPTB may be required in consultation with the specialist concerned • Extension of IP DR-TB EPTB may be required in consultation with the specialist concerned • Refer to guidelines for EPTB duration of treatment		
Pediatric TB	• In children, who are unable to produce sputum, the response to treatment may be assessed clinically. The help if radiological and other relevant investigations may also be taken	Same as above		

Clinical monitoring is the most important criteria for the follow-up of patients with EP DR-TB. Regular patient monitoring and periodic follow-up of nodes and other EP symptoms with culture from the discharging node/sinus are the key in monitoring of treatment in EP lymph nodal DR-TB.

Bacteriological monitoring: Two specimens from the discharging sinus/pus in the lymph node should be collected, one each for smear and culture. The specimen should be taken at the end of the third month of treatment and then every month (at least 30 days apart) in IP till there is pus/discharge from sinus (in the node). Unlike sputum smear and culture, culture from the node can be given only till the pus/discharging sinus is present from the node. The follow-up is mainly based on clinical parameters.

Clinical monitoring: This is important in case of EP DR-TB. Monitoring and follow-up can be done clinically based on the following:
- Weight gain
- Decrease or increase in symptoms (healing of ulcer/scrofuloderma)
- Increase or regression in size of nodes [possibility of Immune Reconstitution Inflammatory Syndrome (IRIS) to be considered and differentiated from disease progression].
- Appearance of new nodes

- If chest symptomatic, monthly sputum for AFB and chest X-ray (to rule out pulmonary involvement).
- Other EP sites to be monitored (USG abdomen, if necessary)
- Serum creatinine—monthly for first three months of treatment and then quarterly till the patient receives Km and further when clinically indicated.
- Liver function test, as clinically indicated
- Monitoring for drug adverse reactions

Same outcome definitions would be used as for pulmonary DR-TB patients. Treatment outcome will depend on availability of culture reports of specimens taken from discharging sinuses, treatment completion, and clinical improvement of the patient.

Management of Contacts of Drug-resistant Tuberculosis

"Close contacts" of DR-TB patients are defined as people living in the same household as the index patient, or spending many hours a day together with the patient in the same indoor space. Contact tracing is an underutilized strategy that can stop the transmission of multidrug-resistant strains. Studies have shown that contact investigation is a high-yield strategy that, in many high-burden TB countries, probably merits more resources even for regular, drug-susceptible TB patients.[13]

All close contacts of DR-TB patients should be identified through contact tracing and evaluated for active TB disease as per RNTCP guidelines.

If the contact is found to be suffering from pulmonary TB disease, irrespective of the smear-based microbiological confirmation, she/he will be identified as a "Presumptive DR-TB." The patient will be initiated on regimen for new or previously treated patient based on their history of previous anti-TB treatment. Simultaneously, two sputum specimens will be transported for culture and DST to an RNTCP-certified C-DST laboratory where she/he will be evaluated as per DR-TB diagnostic algorithm.

If the patient is confirmed as having DR-TB, appropriate DR-TB treatment must be initiated. Further, the patient will be sent to the DDR-TBC ward for pretreatment assessment and initiation of appropriate regimen. Among asymptomatic contacts of patients with DR-TB, it would be important to rule out active TB by appropriate clinical examination and investigation. Although alternative prophylaxis treatments have been suggested, there is no consensus regarding the choice of drug(s) and the duration of treatment. Prompt treatment of DR-TB in index case is the most effective way of preventing the spread of infection to others. There are multiple opportunities to investigate contacts of DR-TB patients, namely:

- *Patient*: Contact investigation starts with education of the DR-TB patient. Patients should be educated about the infectiousness of their disease and the high-risk of transmission to contacts who share the same living space. While they should not be unduly alarmed, they should be informed that their family members are likely already infected with DR-TB, so the most important intervention is to monitor them closely for symptoms of active TB.
- *Family*: One of the most important reasons to do a home visit for every DR-TB patient at the initiation of DR-TB treatment is to do contact investigation. A community nurse or healthcare provider should educate the family that they are all likely already infected with DR-TB, and explain the importance of notifying the community or clinical team quickly about family members who develop symptoms of active TB.
- *Clinical team*: The clinical team has multiple opportunities to inquire about the health of the DR-TB patient's family contacts. At every clinical evaluation, doctors and nurses should ask the patient whether any family member has developed TB symptoms.

- *Community nurses or healthcare providers educated on DR-TB*: During home visits to check adherence or assess the social situation, the community nurse should enquire if there are any family members who have developed symptoms of active TB. The community nurse may directly interview family members at their home as they are best suited to address fears or doubts about the health system or other social barriers to treatment for DR-TB contacts.
- *Community health workers*: In community-based programs that incorporate home-based treatment support, community health workers are the closest to the family and are most likely to identify family members with TB symptoms. This is particularly true for members of the extended family who visit periodically. The following measures should be taken to prevent spread of DR-TB infection:
  - Early diagnosis and appropriate treatment of DR-TB patients.
  - Counseling patient and family on infection control measures such as cough etiquette and sputum disposal.
  - Screening of contacts as per RNTCP guidelines.
  - Further research into effective and nontoxic chemoprophylaxis in areas of high DR-TB prevalence.

Management of Contacts of Drug-resistant Tuberculosis

All individuals who are presumptive TB or presumptive DR-TB are required to have a sputum or an appropriate EP specimen examination for diagnosis. The comprehensive request form for examination of biological specimen for TB is to be used for requesting for microscopy, CBNAAT or culture DST, or chest X-ray or TST, or any other tests. It is essential to record patient details, reason for testing, and type of tests requested. The front page of the form is for recording patient details, reason for testing (diagnosis or follow-up), test requested, result of sputum smear microscopy and NIKSHAY ID (expected in case of notified TB patient subjected for DR-TB screening). This form should be filled by the staff of the health facility that is sending the specimen with a request for examination and expected to be transported along with specimen to the concerned laboratory or health facility for the requested test. Back page is to report the results of CBNAAT, LPA, DST, and any other tests requested.

For all specimens sent from peripheral health institutes, test requests should be initiated from the specimen collecting health facility and entered in NIKSHAY/e-NIKSHAY on the spot in real time. This will enable instant online intimation about the upcoming specimen at the health facility (CBNAAT site or C-DST laboratory) where these tests are requested prior to receipt of the specimen while it is in transit. The result will be updated at the testing health facility in NIKSHAY/e-NIKSHAY on real time to save time required to scan results and send it to the concerned health facility. Final report of the test may be printed out through NIKSHAY at any health facility. Real-time data entry helps the program to disseminate information at all levels such as N/DDR-TBC, district, TU, and PHI to initiate reflex actions for further patient management on real-time basis.

RNTCP Laboratory Register for Culture, CBNAAT, and Drug-susceptibility Testing

The RNTCP laboratory register for culture, CBNAAT, and DST is used to record CBNAAT, LPA, and culture and DST examination results. This will be maintained by the concerned laboratory staff. Results of all specimens tested at these sites are expected to be entered in NIKSHAY/e-NIKSHAY. For all presumptive DR-TB patients, test results should be updated in existing NIKSHAY ID to maintain continuity while presumptive TB patients tested at these laboratories, NIKSHAY ID may be generated, after ensuring that it is not generated elsewhere. The individual should be notified if diagnosed with TB and NIKSHAY ID should be shared with along with the report. Results of subsequent tests carried out will be entered in the same ID. This gives an opportunity to easily extract the test results of all specimen provided by the patient and thereby track his/her response to the treatment. All the follow-up investigations carried out will be entered periodically using the same NIKSHAY ID.

RNTCP PMDT Referral for Treatment Form

The RNTCP PMDT referral for treatment form has to be filled for all confirmed DR-TB patients that are referred from one center to another. The form has to be filled by the doctor of the referring center in duplicate and one copy sent along with the copy of the current treatment card to the referred center. This form can be used for referring the patient at various points in time during the management of the patient between the PHI, DTC, and DR-TBC for reasons such as initiation of treatment, adverse drug reaction, transfer out, ambulatory treatment, or any other reason. In patients that are transferred out, a copy of the updated PMDT treatment card must be sent along with the referral for treatment form.

Referral module in NIKSHAY facilitates access to patient information through NIKSHAY ID. Provision of shifting of patient from one district to another is possible if the patient has changed his/her residence permanently. In NIKSHAY, the referring health facility must update details under "request for transfer" section to intimate receiving health facility about the transfer even before the patient reaches. In addition to information mentioned in "request for transfer" section, the receiving health facility is able to access all other patient information as well. The accountability of transferred patient is now with the receiving health facility and the treatment initiating facility.

RNTCP PMDT Treatment Card

The RNTCP PMDT treatment card is a key instrument for the treatment supporter administrating drugs daily to the patient. The card will be initiated at D/NDR-TBC when the patient is initiated on treatment either on outpatients or on indoor basis. The original treatment card will be maintained at the respective DR-TBC and copy kept by the treatment supporter. The card should be updated daily, documenting the administration of drugs by the treatment supporter. The card is the source to update periodically the PMDT register and adherence details on NIKSHAY. Accountable systems have to be developed locally for updating cards at all levels. When or if the patient moves from DR-TBC to his/her district of residence a copy of the card, must follow the patient. Once the patient has switched to other regimen at NDR-TBC, a new set of treatment cards along with new treatment booklet should be prepared for the patient and the same shared with the field. A copy of this card may be used as a notification form and to inform final outcome of treatment.

Newer Information and Communication Technology (ICT) solutions [Medication Event Reminder Monitor System (MERM), etc.] to promote information management about the patient's treatment adherence are being tested at field level for DR-TB patients. This will help in autoupdation of treatment adherence details in NIKSHAY/e-NIKSHAY as well as flag patients with frequent treatment interruptions to prompt visits of healthcare providers and supervisors to intervene and retrieve the patient on treatment. If the patient is under the ICT monitoring system, treatment card in hard copy should be maintained at the treatment supporter level. A treatment supporter will be relieved from the regular updation of treatment card in NIKSHAY during such condition.

The card contains the following sections:
- *Page 1 of the treatment card*:
  - *Basic demographic information*: Name, sex, age, address, telephone number, state, DR-TBC, district, TU, PHI, and details of the treatment supporter. Some part of this information will be auto populated from available information while other information can be added at district or N/DDR-TBC level which should be supplemented by treating PHI.
- *PMDT TB number*: This is a new unique patient identification number given to the patient at the DR-TBC on initiation of treatment. The PMDT TB number should include S. No/Nodal or District/Name of DR-TBC code/year of initiation of treatment, e.g., PMDT-TB number of first patient started on treatment at Nagpur DDR-TBC during 2017 will be 1/D-NGP/2017. Every year PMDT TB number will be started at 1. The Nodal DR-TB center will maintain its PMDT number separately starting from 1st of every year, e.g., PMDT number of 1st patient initiated at Nodal DR-TBC belong to Nagpur District will be 1/N-NGP/2017. The district where the Nodal DR-TBC is located has to maintain separate District DR-TB PMDT register if center is also functioning as DDR-TBC. This would remain as a transitory system till the time most DR-TB patients are tracked with the help of NIKSHAY. This will be done till it is time to completely transition from paper-based registers to autogeneration of electronic registers from NIKSHAY PMDT modules directly.
- *NIKSHAY ID*: NIKSHAY ID refers to the unique ID which is generated at the time of testing for TB. As per RNTCP Technical and Operational Guidelines (TOG), all TB patients are to be notified at the time of diagnosis. This information is recorded in the TB notification register. Pool of all DR-TB patients (RR/MDR/H Mono/poly, etc.) diagnosed either at CBNAAT laboratory or C-DST laboratories or in private laboratory will be updated digitally. The NIKSHAY ID will capture all subsequent events that are taking place for diagnostic and treatment pathways. This creates a lifecycle approach where multiple events happen for a single patient pertaining to diagnosis and treatment pathways which are captured in a single NIKSHAY ID. All relevant information of a particular patient would be available with the same NIKSHAY ID which can be printed at all accessible users' levels. Once the patient is initiated on treatment, details are captured in PMDT treatment register that is maintained at D/NDR-TBC and PMDT number is assigned. The NIKSHAY ID has a provision to capture more than one PMDT number generated at different D/NDR-TBC while patient transfer is done. This provides a log of patient information that helps in tracking all updates starting from DR-TB diagnosis to long-term treatment outcomes.
- *Reason for testing*: This section lists and describes details of the reason for testing. This includes types of patient that have to be ticked as applicable for new, previously treated, presumptive TB, private referral, presumptive nontuberculous mycobacteria (NTM), criteria for presumptive DR-TB, presumptive H mono/poly and criteria for presumptive XDR-TB.
- *DST results at diagnosis:*
  - Detailed DST information for each patient is captured with date of specimen collection. All DST results for CBNAAT, LPA, and LC-DST are captured here once the result is received. SL-LPA result is available as FQ and/or SLI class resistance.

Resistance is captured as R against all drugs that belong to that group. Once LC-DST result is available, it is mentioned in lower section of DST preferably.
- *HIV testing*: This section lists the date of testing, PID number, date of starting CPT, and ART (wherever applicable). As per the national policy, information sharing on HIV status of patients should be restricted within healthcare facilities based on the concept of "shared confidentiality." Hence, this information must not be written on the copy of the card held by the treatment supporter and patient booklet.
- *Contact tracing*: This section details number of household contacts screened, number of presumptive TB patients identified, number of presumptive TB patients evaluated, number diagnosed with TB, and number of DR-TB diagnosed. First contact screening should be carried out at the time of treatment initiation, however, this should be a continuous process during the course of treatment as any close contact may present with TB symptoms at any point of time during the course of treatment for index patients. In pediatric DR-TB patients, reverse contact tracing to search for an adult index patient in the household must be considered by healthcare workers.

NIKSHAY

NIKSHAY is the platform for the National Tuberculosis Programme Surveillance System. It envisages establishing ICT-enabled state-of-art surveillance system with system utilization by 100% stakeholders, ensuring 100% notification of TB patients at diagnosis (microbiologically confirmed and clinically diagnosed). The program envisions continuous monitoring and treatment adherence for all TB patients registered with e-NIKSHAY, enabling tracking of all registered TB patients across TB elimination life cycle, geographies, transfers, and referrals.

The first step is to ensure complete entry in all formats. Dashboard functions to track activities and online monitoring indicators with graphical and geomapping displays in NIKSHAY/e-NIKSHAY is helpful in program monitoring provided completeness of data entered is ascertained. Primarily, the source of information for all monitoring indicators will be NIKSHAY. Thus validation of actual report and the entered report should be done at each level to sustain quality of information available digitally. Patient-wise details and aggregated monitoring indicators for specified period is available within NIKSHAY.

e-NIKSHAY

In an attempt to reduce the TB burden in the country, it is envisaged that an ICT system such as e-NIKSHAY could help with coordinated planning and action that is required at various levels. This would be from improving patient awareness and ease of access to TB care to time-bound and effective diagnosis and treatment by the service providers. The goal would be to develop a common integrated platform as an open system to engage ecosystem stakeholders toward effective, timely, and quality assured diagnosis and effective treatment of TB. It would essentially use a case-based approach to the TB lifecycle, enabling patient-based tracking and monitoring allowing for stakeholder integration, as well as timely and accurate reporting and real-time decision support.

The RNTCP shall roll out e-NIKSHAY with support to states on logistics and trainings. This platform will serve as a web-based, case-based recording and reporting system which will also feed into routine surveillance of DR-TB in the country. e-NIKSHAY will be rolled out initially in the states of Gujarat and Maharashtra and gradually scaled up nationally by end of 2018.

Role of e-NIKSHAY in Recording, Reporting, and SME (Supervision, Monitoring, and Evaluation)

- e-NIKSHAY will gradually replace the cumbersome paper-based system of recording and reporting. Options shall be provided to capture the event at origin through provision of mobile/web applications, tablets, and call centers on real-time basis. This will change and improve reporting structures for more agility and efficiency by providing relevant reports at relevant levels without delay due to paper-based collection, collation, and compilation of reports.
- e-NIKSHAY will generate user-specific task lists on real-time basis according to their job responsibilities aiding staff to prioritize tasks at various levels. ICT-enabled adherence mechanisms [99 Directly observed treatment, short-course (DOTS), MERM, etc.] will feed treatment-related information from patients and providers into e-NIKSHAY enriching it as a patient care and support platform to prioritize patients for differential care.
- e-NIKSHAY will aid the referral and feedback mechanism under the program by providing real-time information on referral of patients for treatment initiation and ADR management. This will aid the program to manage referral and provide feedbacks thereby decreasing lost to follow-up and improved tracking of patients nationally.
- e-NIKSHAY will populate dashboards for all supervisory staff at various levels to aid in their day-to-day work by providing dashboards for different facilities, categories of staff, and geographies. This will aid supervisors and program managers in identifying areas, both thematic and functional for intensive supervision.
- e-NIKSHAY shall generate interactive tables of real-time monitoring indicators to aid review at various levels. The platform will generate alerts in the form of SMS, e-mails, and call from call centers for patients, providers, and supervisors for actions to promote favorable outcomes and improve program management efficiency. The indicators shall be projected as interactive tables/maps to promote information-driven monitoring at all levels.

INFECTION CONTROL MEASURES

Evidence indicates that DR-TB is similar in transmissibility to DS-TB. Thus, infection control policies and strategies are not much different for DR-TB. All facilities treating DR-TB patients must comply with adequate infection control measures. Ensuring implementation of infection control policy in all healthcare facilities, at public/private/household level and in congregate settings (correctional facilities, military barracks, homeless shelters, refugee camps, student dormitories and nursing homes, among others) is essential. This will help prevent transmission before diagnosis up to initial stages of treatment till the patient has culture converted and turned noninfectious. Actions are required at national and subnational levels to provide managerial direction and at health facility level to implement AIC measures.

Objectives of Revised National Tuberculosis Control Programme

- Achievement of at least 85% cure rate of infectious cases of TB through DOTS involving peripheral health functionaries Augmentation of case-finding activities through quality sputum microscopy to detect at least 70% of estimated cases

The vision of RNTCP is that the people suffering from TB receive the highest standards of care and support from all healthcare providers of their choice. It is spelt out in the National Strategic Plan (2012-17) to extend the umbrella of quality TB care and control to include those provided by the private sector.

Revised National Tuberculosis Control Programme-endorsed Tuberculosis diagnostics

- Smear microscopy for acid-fast bacilli
  - Sputum smear stained with Ziehl–Neelsen staining or
  - Fluorescence stains and examined under direct or indirect microscopy with or without LED.
- Culture
  - Solid (LJ) media or
  - Liquid media (Middlebrook) using manual semiautomatic or automatic machines, e.g., Bactec, MGIT
- Rapid diagnostic molecular test
  - Conventional PCR-based LPA for MTB complex
  - Real-time PCR-based Nu NAAT for MTB complex e.g., GeneXpert
- Radiography where available
- Tuberculin skin test

Ban on TB serology: The serological tests are based on antibody response, which is highly variable in TB and may reflect remote infection rather than active disease. Currently available serological tests are having poor specificity and should not be used for the diagnosis of pulmonary or extra pulmonary TB. Their import, manufacturing, sale, distribution, and use is banned by the Government of India.

REFERENCES

1. Central TB Division, Directorate General of Health Services, Ministry of Health & Family Welfare, Government of India. (2017). TB India 2017. [online] Available from https://tbcindia.gov.in/WriteReadData/TB%20India%202017.pdf. [Last accessed January, 2020].
2. Central TB Division, Directorate General of Health Services, Ministry of Health & Family Welfare, Government of India. (2012). Guidelines on Programmatic Management of Drug Resistant TB in India. [online] Available from https://tbcindia.gov.in/index1.php?lang=1&level=2&sublinkid=4780&lid=3306. [Last accessed January, 2020]., New Delhi, 2012.
3. Central TB Division, Directorate General of Health Services, Ministry of Health & Family Welfare, Government of India. (2017). National Strategic Plan 2017-25 for TB Elimination in India. [online]. Available from https://tbcindia.gov.in/WriteReadData/NSP%20Draft%2020.02.2017%201.pdf. [Last accessed January, 2020].
4. Central TB Division, Directorate General of Health Services, Ministry of Health & Family Welfare, Government of India. (2016). Guidelines for Use of Bedaquiline in RNTCP through conditional access under PMDT in India. [online] Available from https://tbcindia.gov.in/index1.php?lang=1&level=2&sublinkid=4682&lid=3248. [Last accessed January, 2020].
5. Central TB Division, Directorate General of Health Services, Ministry of Health & Family Welfare, Government of India. (2016). RNTCP Technical and Operational Guidelines for TB Control in India. [online] Available from https://tbcindia.gov.in/index1.php?sublinkid=4573&level=2&lid=3177&lang=1. [Last accessed January, 2020].
6. National TB Institute, Bangalore & Central TB Division, Directorate General of Health Services, Ministry of Health & Family Welfare, Government of India. First National Tuberculosis Drug Resistance Survey in India. (2014-2016). [online]. Available from https://tbcindia.gov.in/showfile.php?lid=3315. [Last accessed January, 2020].

7. World Health Organization. (2016). The use of molecular line probe assays for the detection of resistance to second-line antituberculosis drugs.[online] Available from https://apps.who.int/iris/handle/10665/246131. [Last accessed January, 2020].
8. World Health Organization. (2015). Implementing Tuberculosis Diagnostics - Policy Framework. [online] Available from https://www.who.int/tb/publications/implementing_TB_diagnostics/en/. [Last accessed January, 2020].
9. World Health Organization. (2016). WHO treatment guidelines for drug-resistant tuberculosis. . [online] Available from https://apps.who.int/iris/bitstream/handle/10665/250125/9789241549639-webannexes-eng.pdf. [Last accessed January, 2020].
10. World Health Organization. (2013). The use of bedaquiline in the treatment of multi-drug resistant tuberculosis - Interim policy guidance. [online] Available from https://www.who.int/tb/publications/mdrtb-treatment-guideline/en/. [Last accessed January, 2020].
11. World Health Organization. (2014). The use of delamanid in the treatment of multidrug-resistant tuberculosis - Interim policy guidance. [online] Available from https://www.who.int/tb/publications/Delamanid_interim_policy/en/. [Last accessed January, 2020].
12. World Health Organization. (2016). Report of the Guideline Development Group Meeting on the use of bedaquiline in the treatment of multidrug-resistant tuberculosis - A review of available evidence (2016). [online] Available from https://apps.who.int/iris/handle/10665/254712. [Last accessed January, 2020].
13. Morrison J, Pai M, Hopewell PC. Tuberculosis and latent tuberculosis infection in close contacts of people with pulmonary tuberculosis in low-income and middle-income countries: a systematic review and meta-analysis. Lancet Infect Dis. 2008;8(6):359-68.

CHAPTER 3

Pathology of Tuberculosis in the Genitourinary Tract

Anila Abraham Kurien

GRANULOMA

The classical hallmark lesion in tuberculosis is an epithelioid granuloma (**Fig. 1**). The granuloma creates an immune microenvironment in which the infection can be contained. A typical granuloma is composed of epithelioid cells, Langhans giant cells, and lymphocytes surrounding a central region of caseous necrosis.

Epithelioid cells are activated macrophages, which develop an epithelial-cell-like appearance. On hematoxylin and eosin (H&E) stained sections, the epithelioid cells have indistinct cell boundaries and abundant pale pink cytoplasm.

Epithelioid cells fuse to form Langhans giant cells. These giant cells have 20 or more nuclei arranged in the periphery in a horse shoe pattern or as clusters of nuclei at the two poles of the giant cells (**Fig. 2**). Although traditional Langhans cells were associated with tuberculosis (TB), they are not specific for TB. They can be found in all types of granulomatous disease, including sarcoidosis, syphilis, leprosy, and fungal infections.

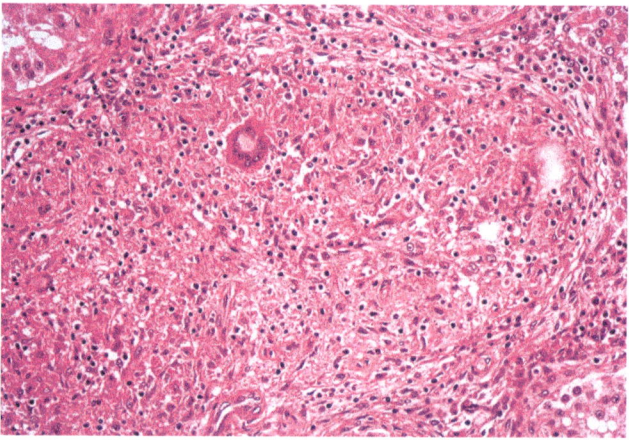

FIG. 1: An epithelioid granuloma in the testis. Central caseous necrosis may not be seen in all granulomas.

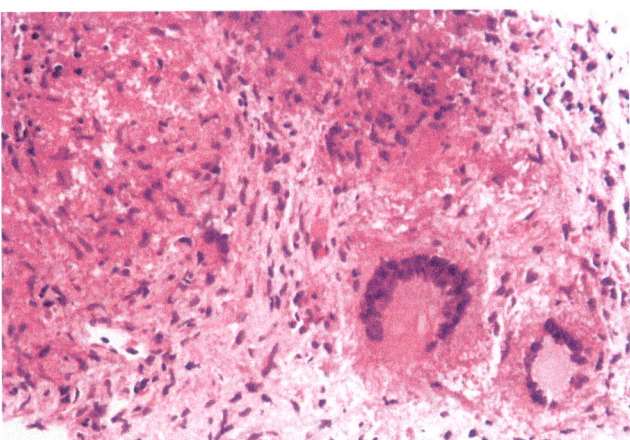

FIG. 2: Multinucleated giant cells of the Langhans type.

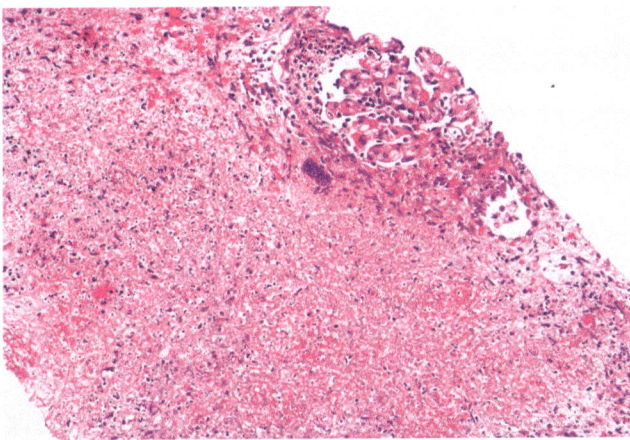

FIG. 3: The image shows a large area of caseous necrosis destroying the renal parenchyma.

Caseous necrosis is a unique form of necrosis where the necrotic material resembles soft cheese. On H&E stained sections, they appear as pink amorphous material (**Fig. 3**). Unlike in coagulative necrosis where the histologic architecture is preserved, the tissue architecture is completely destroyed in caseous necrosis. Not all tubercular granulomas show central caseous necrosis. Also, caseous necrosis can also be seen in syphilis and in fungal infections like histoplasmosis, cryptococcosis, and coccidioidomycosis.

A typical granuloma has four zones.
1. Central caseous necrosis.
2. Epithelioid macrophages, Langhans giant cells, and lymphocytes form the inner cellular zone.
3. Plasma cells, lymphocytes, and macrophages form the outer cellular zone.
4. Rim of fibrous tissue.

The granulomas may contain viable mycobacteria, which are seen in the inner cellular zone. The central necrotic zone does not favor the growth of the bacteria as it has low pH, low oxygen tension, and high levels of fatty acids.[1]

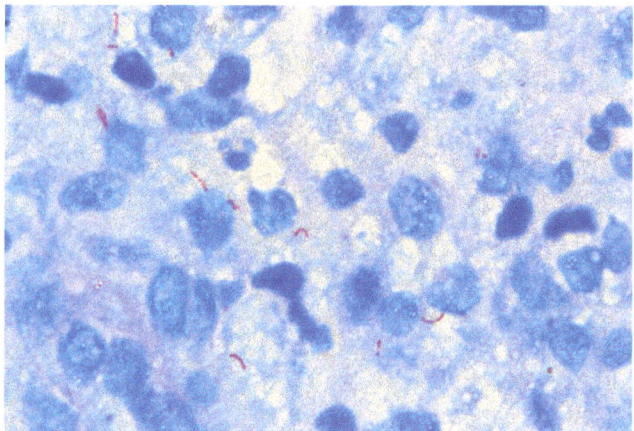

FIG. 4: Acid-fast bacilli are clearly visible on Ziehl–Neelsen stain.

HISTOCHEMICAL STAINS TO IDENTIFY MYCOBACTERIA

Mycobacteria have a waxy cell well composed of *mycolic* acid. This acid makes them "acid-fast" which means that the bacteria will retain stains (it is resistant to decolorization) even after the treatment with an acid. Acid fastness is a unique characteristic of mycobacteria and this property is used in its detection in infected tissue.

Histochemical stains used in pathologic specimens to identify mycobacteria:
- Ziehl–Neelsen (ZN) stain using bright field microscopy (**Fig. 4**).
- Auramine stain using fluorescence microscopy.

In persons with intact cell-mediated immunity, the bacilli are contained within the granuloma and the granuloma undergoes fibrosis and sometimes calcification. Some bacilli survive inside the granuloma for a long time in a dormant state. In about 10% of these individuals, the bacilli will reactivate and the granuloma is unable to contain the bacteria. The caseous necrosis undergoes liquefaction and the outer fibrous tissue loss its structural integrity. There is destruction of the adjacent tissue. The semi liquid necrotic material in the center of the granuloma drains out and a cavity is formed.

In an immunosuppressed individual, the granulomas are less well formed and caseous necrosis is less frequently present. Mycobacteria are more easily identified in these lesions.

When the immunosuppression is severe or when the infection is caused by one of the atypical bacteria like *Mycobacterium avium-intracellulare*, no granulomas may be identified. The lesion consists of sheets of macrophages with abundant pale cytoplasm. Caseous necrosis is not a feature in these lesions. Mycobacteria are packed within the macrophages and are easily identified by histochemical stains.[1]

TUBERCULOSIS OF THE KIDNEY

Kidney may be involved as a part of disseminated generalized infection or as a disease localized to the genitourinary tract.[2-8]

Gross and Microscopic Examination

As Part of Disseminated Infection

Millet sized (2–3 mm) yellowish white lesions are seen throughout the renal parenchyma with the periglomerular area in the renal cortex being densely involved.

On microscopic examination, these lesions consist of epithelioid granuloma with or without central necrosis.

Mycobacteria can usually be identified in these granulomas but sometime are difficult to find.[2,3]

As A Localized Infection

Localized renal tuberculosis usually presents as a unilateral lesions. However, autopsy studies have demonstrated that they are commonly bilateral.
Localized infection in the renal parenchyma has three morphological appearances.[3]
1. Pseudotumor/mass lesion
2. Pyelonephritis
3. Interstitial nephritis

Pseudotumor/Mass Lesion

- The pseudotumor like mass lesion consists of multiple coalescing epithelioid granuloma with large central necrosis causing local tissue destruction (**Fig. 5**). Large *cavitary* lesions develop when the necrotic tissue drain out.
- The inflammation can extend outside the renal capsule as a mass lesion.
- The granuloma can damage the blood supply to the renal papillae and cause necrosis and sloughing of the renal papillae.[5]

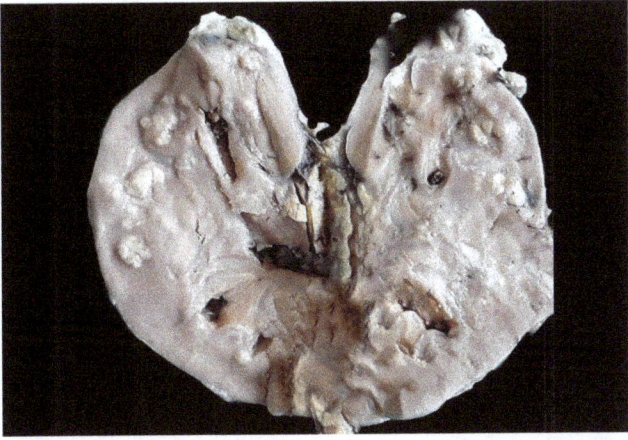

FIG. 5: Tuberculosis of the kidney. There are multiple caseating granulomas forming mass lesions. Caseating lymph nodes are seen at the hilum.

Tuberculous Pyelonephritis
- The granulomatous inflammation may disrupt the renal tubules.
- The bacilli thus gains entry into the collecting system and renal pelvis.
- They can progress to localized or generalized pyonephrosis also known as "cement" or "putty" kidney.[2,4]
- Many cases of tuberculosis pyelonephritis progress to end stage kidney damage.
- The kidney appears small and shrunken and the cortex is markedly thinned out.
- Dystrophic calcification is seen in the collecting system.[2-6]

Tuberculous Interstitial Nephritis
- The kidneys appear normal in size with smooth contours on gross examination.
- No mass lesions are seen on serial sectioning of the kidney.[3]
- Microscopic examination reveals interstitial inflammation with epithelioid granuloma that is usually noncaseating (**Fig. 6**).
- Occasional foci of caseous necrosis may be identified.
- Mycobacteria are usually not identified on ZN staining.[6]

Differential Diagnosis
- Sarcoidosis
- Drug-induced interstitial nephritis
- Fungal infections
    - They are associated with tissue destruction and necrosis. Caseating granulomas are seen. Histochemical stains for fungi and acid-fast bacilli help establish the diagnosis.
- Xanthogranulomatous pyelonephritis
    - Sheets of foamy macrophages infiltrate the renal parenchyma, ill-defined granuloma may be seen. No discrete granuloma formation or caseous necrosis is identified.[2,3,5]

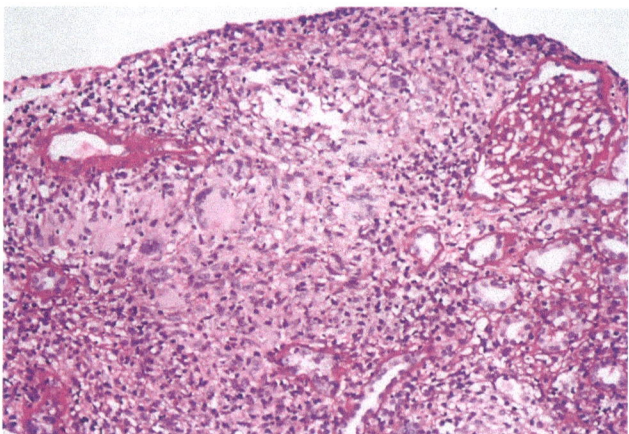

FIG. 6: Tuberculous granulomatous interstitial nephritis. Multiple noncaseating granulomas are seen in the interstitium of the kidney.

TUBERCULOSIS OF THE PELVIS AND URETER

- Tuberculosis involves the renal pelvis and ureter as a part of direct spread from the kidney.
- The granulomatous inflammation produces ureteric strictures.
- The ureter appears irregular with segmental dilatation alternating with areas of stricture.
- This causes obstruction and/or reflux.[2,3,5,7]

TUBERCULOSIS OF THE BLADDER

- The vast majority of cases of TB bladder arises from direct extension from the kidney.[2,5]
- Tuberculous cystitis can also occur as a result of spread from the epididymis.
- Local instillation of BCG for the medication of urothelial carcinoma in situ and superficial bladder cancer can cause granulomatous cystitis.[8]

Gross Examination

In the cases where the infection arises from the kidney, the mucosa near the ureteric orifice is involved first.

In advanced cases, the disease spreads to involve the entire bladder. The bladder becomes small and contracted.

Fistulas may rarely develop.[2,5]

Microscopic Examination

Microscopic appearance of lesion caused by BCG is identical to those seen in the classical infectious disease. Foci of caseation may be present and mycobacteria may be identified on special stains.[8]

Differential Diagnosis

Post-biopsy/Resection Granuloma

Found in about 3% of patients with post biopsy/resection and in 13.6% of patients who had at least two surgical procedures. Seen as necrotizing and palisading granuloma which heals with scarring. They occur as a local reaction to tissue necrosis caused by surgery and/or cautery.[9]

TUBERCULOSIS OF THE PROSTATE

Tuberculous involvement of the prostate is usually the result of hematogenous dissemination of the bacteria from the site of primary infection. It can also occur as a part of local spread form the genital tract. Rarely, tuberculous involvement of the prostate has been reported following intravesical BCG therapy. Sexual transmission is extremely rare.[2,10,11]

Gross Appearance

- The prostate appears firm to hard and nodular.
- It may or may not be enlarged.

- Dense fibrotic nodules may be seen on serial sectioning.
- Tuberculous lesions are usually located in the peripheral region and lateral lobes of the prostate.
- Foci of caseous necrosis may be seen.
- It can cause cavitation and sloughing.
- Rare cases of autoprostatectomy have been reported.
- Abscess formation may be seen in severely immunosuppressed patients.

Microscopic Appearance

Microscopic examination shows epithelioid granulomas with or without central caseous necrosis.

These granulomas are usually diffused and are not confined to the periductal or periglomerular region.

Differential Diagnosis

- Nonspecific granulomatous prostatitis
  It is the most common granulomatous inflammatory condition in the prostate and it accounts for greater than half the cases with granulomatous inflammation in the prostate. It is a self-limiting benign condition and usually an incidental finding. It occurs due to the blockage with disruption and damage of prostatic ducts. The cell debris and prostatic secretions from within the blocked ducts leak into the surrounding stroma and elicit a granulomatous reaction. These granulomas are typically noncaseous and poorly defined and centered around damaged ducts and acini. Eosinophils and neutrophils may be seen. It is important to differentiate nonspecific granulomatous prostatitis from tuberculous prostatitis as the former requires no specific treatment.[11]
- Infectious agents
  Treponema pallidum, viruses, and various fungi can produce granulomatous inflammation of the prostate. Histochemical stains like Periodic acid–Schiff (PAS), Gömöri methenamine silver (GMS), and ZN stains are helpful to identify the etiology.[10]

TUBERCULOSIS OF THE EPIDIDYMIS AND TESTIS

Tuberculous epididymitis results from retrograde extension from the prostate as well as from hematogenous spread. Retrograde spread following intravesical BCG therapy has been reported.

Isolated tuberculous orchitis without epididymal involvement is rare. It usually occurs as a result of contiguous extension from the epididymis.[2,12,13]

Gross Examination

About 30–40% of tuberculous epididymitis is bilateral.

The earliest lesion appears as yellowish necrotic areas in the tail of the epididymis. The tail of the epididymis is usually involved first because of its rich blood supply and also because it is the first portion to be involved by urinary reflux.

As the disease progresses, it involves the entire epididymis and extends into the testis and presents as a necrotic scrotal mass which on gross examination can mimic a testicular tumor (**Fig. 7**).

Scrotal abscess formation or scrotal sinus formation can be seen in advanced cases.[2,12]

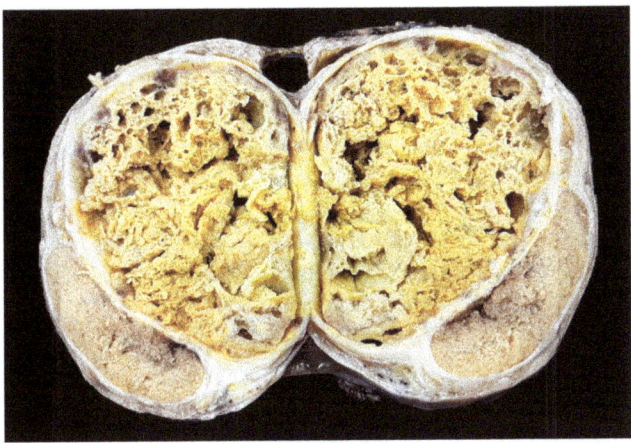

FIG. 7: Tuberculous epididymo-orchitis presenting as a necrotic mass in the scrotum.

Microscopic Examination

Multiple epithelioid granuloma replaces the normal tissue. Areas of fibrosis may be seen between the granuloma. Extensive tissue destruction with large areas of caseous necrosis is common.

Differential Diagnosis

- Idiopathic granulomatous orchitis
  A benign condition due to an autoimmune reaction to spermatogenic elements. Epithelioid granulomatous reaction is seen confined to seminiferous tubules, along with extensive interstitial lymphoplasmacytic inflammation. Well-formed granulomas and caseous necrosis are usually not seen. Special stains for mycobacteria and fungi are negative.[14,15]
- Pyogenic epididymo orchitis
  Resembles granulomatous orchitis, usually caused by *Escherichia coli*.[16]
- Leprosy
  Though rare, testicular involvement is thought to be due to the lower temperature of scrotum. Numerous acid-fast bacilli laden macrophages are seen in the perivascular regions. No well-formed granuloma or caseous necrosis is seen. Dense fibrosis replaces the normal tissue as the disease advances.[17]
- Granulomatous orchitis due to brucellosis
  Seminiferous tubules and interstitium infiltrated by granulomas of non-necrotizing type. Inflammatory infiltrate is rich in plasma cells.[15]
- *Histoplasma capsulatum*
  Can present as a scrotal mass with caseating granuloma, and giant cells. PAS, GMS, and ZN stain helps establish the diagnosis.[18]

HIV AND GENITOURINARY TUBERCULOSIS

Tuberculosis is the most frequent opportunistic infection in patients infected with HIV. It has been reported that infection with HIV is associated with a higher risk for extrapulmonary involvement. Tuberculosis can occur in any phase of the HIV infection, often before a significant drop in CD4$^+$ T-cell counts occur or other clinical features suggestive of HIV infection or AIDS appear.[19]

Patients with tuberculosis and HIV present at a younger age than patients without HIV infection. They also more often present with fever, fatigue, bacteremia, diffuse pulmonary disease, lymph node disease, and disseminated tuberculosis with genitourinary tract involvement.[20]

Histopathological examination reveals diffuse lesions with extensive tissue necrosis, few or no mature epithelioid cells and numerous tubercle bacilli. Secondary bacterial and mycotic infections and abscess formation are common.[19]

REFERENCES

1. Shah KK, Pritt BS, Alexander MP. Histopathologic review of granulomatous inflammation. Journal of clinical tuberculosis and other mycobacterial diseases. 2017;7: 1-12.
2. Wise GJ, Marella VK. Genitourinary manifestation of tuberculosis. Urol Clin North Am. 2003;30:111-21.
3. Eastwood JB, Corbishley CM, Grange J. Tuberculosis and the kidney. J Am Soc Nephrol. 2001;12:1307-14.
4. Najar MS, Bhat MA, Wani IA, Banday KA, Reshi AR, Daga BA, et al . Profile of renal tuberculosis in 63 patients. Indian J Nephrol. 2003;13:104-7.
5. Kapoor R, Ansari MS, Mandhani A, Gulia A. Clinical presentation and diagnostic approach in cases of genitourinary tuberculosis. Indian J Urol. 2008;24(3):401–5.
6. Merchant S, Bharati A, Merchant N. Tuberculosis of the genitourinary system-Urinary tract tuberculosis: Renal tuberculosis-Part I. Indian J Radiol Imaging 2013;23:46-63.
7. Daher Ede F, da Silva GB Jr, Barros EJ. Renal tuberculosis in the modern era. Am J Trop Med Hyg. 2013;88(1):54–64.
8. Gonzalez OY, Musher DM, Brar I, et al. Spectrum of Bacille Calmette-Guerin (BCG) infection after intravesical BCG immunotherapy. CID. 2003;36: 140-8.
9. Spagnolo, DV, Waring PM.Bladder granulomata after bladder surgery. Am J Clin Pathol.1986;86(1): 430–437.
10. Gupta N, Mandal AK, Singh SK. Tuberculosis of the prostate and urethra: a review. Indian J Urol. 2008;24(3):388–91.
11. Shukla P, Gulwani HV, Kaur S. Granulomatous prostatitis: clinical and histomorphologic survey of the disease in a tertiary care hospital. Prostate Int. 2017;5(1):29-34.
12. Stein AL, Miller DB. Tuberculous epididymo-orchitis: a case report. J Urol 1983;129:613.
13. Viswaroop B S, Kekre N, Gopalakrishnan G. Isolated tuberculous epididymitis: A review of forty cases. J Postgrad Med. 2005;51:109-11.
14. Dhand S, Casalino DD. Idiopathic granulomatous orchitis. J Urol. 2011 Oct;186(4):1477-8.
15. Salmeron I, Ramirez-Escobar MA, Puertas F, Marcos R, Garcia-Marcos F, Sanchez R. Granulomatous epididymo-orchitis: sonographic features and clinical outcome in brucellosis, tuberculosis and idiopathic granulomatous epididymo-orchitis.
16. Yang DM, Yoon MH et al. Comparison of tuberculous and pyogenic epididymal abscesses. AJR. 2001;177: 1131-1135.
17. Yadav N, Kar S, Patrick S, Date P, Ramteke K, Manwar P. Secondary azospermia due to leprous involvement of testis- a case report. Fertil Sci Res. 2019;6:49-51.
18. Tichindelean C, East JW, Sarria JC. Disseminated histoplasmosis presenting as granulomatous epididymo-orchitis. 2009;338(3):238-240.
19. Nzerue C, Drayton J, Oster R, Hewan-Lowe K. Genitourinary tuberculosis in patients with HIV infection: clinical features in an inner-city hospital population. Am J Med Sci. 2000;320(5):299-303.
20. Havlir DV and Barnes PF. Tuberculosis in patients with human immunodeficiency virus infection. N Engl J Med . 1999; 340: 367–73
21. Nzerue C et al. Genitourinary tuberculosis in patients with HIV infection: clinical features in an innercity hospital population. Am J Med Sci . 2000;320: 299–303.

CHAPTER 4

Microbiology of Today's Relevance

Camilla Rodrigues, Yash Pamecha

DIAGNOSIS AND MANAGEMENT OF GENITOURINARY TUBERCULOSIS

Indian still does face the problem of genitourinary tuberculosis (GUTB). Out of the 1.8 million cases of tuberculosis (TB), approximately one-fifth are extrapulmonary. In spite of the modern amenities and newer diagnostic modalities, >1,000 people die every day in India. Here, we will be discussing the dilemmas with diagnosis of GUTB.[1-3]

SAMPLE COLLECTION FOR GENITOURINARY TUBERCULOSIS

Urine Samples

The yield of acid-fast bacilli (AFB) in urinary sample is very low because of two reasons. First, urinary Koch's is a paucibacillary disease as it is due to reactivation of latent bacteria in the urinary system. Second, there is intermittent shedding of bacilli in urine. Because of these reasons, it is very important to obtain a good sample for detection of tuberculous bacilli in urine.[4]

Method of Urine Collection

Patient is asked to collect morning first voided urine in a sterile container. He should collect whole of the voided volume for sample. In case where patient has nocturia and goes very frequently, patient is asked to collect all the voided urine from the time after he goes to sleep till the first time he voids in the morning he wakes up.

Storage and Transport of Sample

Storage in a sterile container preferably, at an ambient temperature of about 20–22°C.

The container should be given to the laboratory within 2 hours of voiding. No need to add any preservative chemical or reagent into the container.

Number of Samples

Three samples on different days are sufficient for the microbiologist for detection of *Mycobacterium tuberculosis*.

Fluid Samples
- Urinary samples from bladder has a low yield. Hence, microbiological detection of *M. tuberculosis* is a difficult task.
- Therefore, whenever possible an attempt should be made to collect urine directly from kidney/upper tracts.
- Per cutaneous puncture and aspiration of urine from pelvicalyceal system is the best sample. However, if percutaneous aspiration is not possible, a cystoscopic ureteric lavage with normal saline and aspirate of the ureteric wash is also considered to be a good sample with higher yield as compared to bladder urine.
- Again, as for voided urine, three samples are sufficient and should be stored and transported in a similar way as urine samples.

Tissue Samples
- Tissue from the organs is believed to contain more bacillary load as compared to the fluids sent for microbiological detection. Biopsies should be sent in six different containers filled with normal saline.
- Formalin should not be used if the tissue is to be sent to microbiologist.
- More biopsy can be taken if histopathological analysis is required.
- In such cases, formalin should be used to preserve the specimen.

Decontamination Process
Contamination of voided urine with commensal nontuberculous mycobacteria is a frequent occurrence. Such nontuberculous mycobacteria may also grow in culture and result in contamination.

Once the sample is received in the laboratory, it undergoes treatment with various chemicals to eliminate unwanted commensal nontuberculous mycobacteria which interfere with microbiological test results such as Xpert and mycobacteria growth indicator tube (MGIT).

One of the drawback of this decontamination process is that it eliminates 40% of tuberculous mycobacteria as well along with nontuberculous mycobacteria. This percentage becomes significant for urinary samples as they are already paucibacillary and the yield is low. Hence, it becomes difficult to get microbiological tests positive for urinary samples.

MICROBIOLOGICAL TESTS AVAILABLE FOR DETECTION OF GUTB
For a long time, routine microscopy AFB staining and culture have remained gold standard for the diagnosis of TB.

Newer tests like florescent microscopy and various liquid cultures and drug sensitivity tests are very much needed but being developed gradually.
- *Demonstration of AFB by Ziehl–Neelsen (ZN) staining*: It has been a basic test for all developing countries. Though it is one of the fastest test and essential test, the detection depends upon the skill of the technician and proper approach. It is also inferior to culture procedure.

The diagnostic accuracy can be increased by use of fluorescent staining instead of conventional ZN staining.

However, because urinary and other extrapulmonary samples are paucibacillary with low microbial burden, it is difficult to get the smears positive for diagnosis of GUTB .Hence, it is practical to avoid sending urinary samples for AFB smear if cost is an issue. AFB smear may be useful for aspirates from suspected tuberculous abscess/cavities.

- *Mycobacterial culture in the diagnosis of TB*: The number of bacilli to be detected on staining methods is approximately 1,000/mL and if lesser than this number the chance of finding the bacillus is <10%.

However, a positive culture requires lesser number of bacilli as low as 100/mL and hence the culture is a more sensitive test than staining.

Another disadvantage of staining methods is that it is not able to distinguish between pathogenic and nonpathogenic bacilli as they are morphologically similar. Contamination does decrease the specificity of a culture test too.

- *Molecular approaches for TB diagnosis*:
  - *CBNAAT (cartridge-based nucleic acid amplification test) Xpert M. tuberculosis/ rifampicin (RIF)*: Here, the Cepheid GeneXpert[5] system is used through a molecular automated test to detect *M. tuberculosis* and the presence of RIF resistance. The specific sequence of *rpoB* gene is amplified by heminested real time polymerase chain reaction (PCR) assay and the molecular beacons are used for probing for mutations within the RIF resistance determination region within a short period of 2 hours. Currently this test is not validated for urine specimens.
  - *Polymerase chain reaction[6]:* This test allows for amplification of the gene sequence of deoxyribonucleic acid (DNA) in vitro even if a few number of mycobacteria are present, leading to better rapid visualization and identification of mycobacteria. The target sequence used in this PCR is the insertion sequence IS6110.11.35. This is a sequence specific for *M. tuberculosis* and is used for offering multiple targets for amplification (up to 20 times in the genome). A study from Bangladesh reports the sensitivity and specificity of IS6110 sequence to be 94.7% and 100% respectively. The conclusion of this discussion is "PCR is an excellent rapid method than any of the previous culture methods."

    This test is now available in all Revised National Tuberculosis Control Programme (RNTCP) free of cost.
  - *Pyrosequencing[7]:* It is a useful method for detection of resistance especially in a retreatment case. It is a molecular diagnostic tool for detection of resistance to RIF, isoniazid (INH), ethambutol (EMB), streptomycin (SM), and amikacin (AMK) in TB. The *Mycobacterium* detection rates for RIF, INH, EMB, SM, and AMK are: 95.5%, 79.2%, 70.2%, 70.3%, 84.5%, 96.5%, and 91.1%.

CLINICAL SCENARIOS IN DIAGNOSIS OF GUTB: PRACTICAL TIPS

- Clinical features suspicious of GUTB and the radiological features are suggestive of TB, but microbiological tests negative for TB—here, we can start Category 1 anti-Koch treatment (AKT) without positive microbiology tests.
  - Please note that emphasis is on the clinical suspicion.

- Clinical features are negative, microbiology is negative but radiological features are suggestive of TB—here do not give AKT. Keep the patient in follow-up and collect better samples. Please note that here the specimens can be collected directly from the lesion to improve microbiological detection and should be repeated as required till the diagnosis is established or disproved.
- If only microbiology tests are positive with no clinical and radiological evidence to support, make sure culture is done at a reliable laboratory and whether they have tested for MPT64 antigen in the growth. If MPT64 antigen has not been tested, use the growth in culture vial to test the same. If positive then start AKT. If negative obtain repeat samples.
- Patient with pulmonary tuberculosis (PTB) received/completed Category 1 AKT but now developed extrapulmonary tuberculosis (EPTB) within 6 months to 2 years post completion of treatment then it is a problem as to what should be your next line of management?

Probably this is the same strain of *M. tuberculosis*, now activated in the new organ where it was lying latent, because of immunodeficiency or incomplete treatment. In such cases give another course of Category 1 AKT.

Patient with GUTB received Category 1 AKT, now showing progression in the form of new anatomical lesions such as subcortical abscess or cavity or tubercles what does it suggest?

This is again endogenous reactivation of same strain which can also be termed as relapse. However, reactivation with a mutant strain is more likely if patient has not completed AKT properly.

Start on Category 1 AKT. If it is relapse with same strain it should respond.

Maximum relapse's of TB occur within 6 months to 2 years and usually is with the same strain.

If patient does not respond or is a relapse second time, rule out the possibility of a resistant mutant strain by sending samples for GeneXpert and culture.

Apart from drug resistance, other causes of relapse are poor immunological status or immunocompromised states such as human immunodeficiency virus (HIV), pregnancy, diabetes mellitus (DM). Another reason may be poor penetration of drug at the site of infection.

Gene sequencing is a vital tool to diagnose drug resistance in such patients.

Collect samples for pyrosequencing and start multidrug resistant (MDR) regimen only if culture shows resistance to the first-line drugs.

Multidrug resistant should not be started without culture reports.

DIAGNOSIS OF GENITOURINARY TUBERCULOSIS

Extrapulmonary tuberculosis (EPTB) accounts for approximately 10–20% of all the TB affected population. Genitourinary tuberculosis (GUTB) is the third most common location of EPTB, after pleural and lymph node involvement. In addition, concomitant GUTB and pulmonary TB are found in 2–10% and in 15–20% of patients in developed and developing countries respectively.[8] Twenty percent of EPTB cases reported annually are urinary TB. Due to nonspecific symptoms in GUTB patients, diagnosis is a major challenge especially in resource limited settings. Despite the fact that involvement of genitourinary organs is almost always secondary to TB elsewhere in the body and is rarely

TABLE 4.1: Diagnostic criteria of urinary tuberculosis.[10]

Classification	Definition
Definite urinary TB	Patients fulfill criterion 1 or 2: 1. Clinical suspected cases plus one or more of the following: positive smear microscopy examination; or positive mycobacterial culture examination 2. Clinical suspected cases plus positive pathological examination
Clinically diagnosed urinary TB case	Clinical suspected cases plus the clinical improvement after empirical anti-TB treatment

contagious, GUTB can result in a significant morbidity and even mortality due to renal failure.

Tubercular involvement of the genitourinary organs is almost always secondary to pulmonary infection. This subclinical pulmonary infection leads to hematogenous spread of the TB bacilli in the kidneys, epididymis, prostate, and various other organs of the body. Initially, spread occurs in more vascular parts such as cortex of the kidneys and globus minor of the epididymis, and is bilateral. After immunity develops, these lesions cicatrize in about 6 months or so and a latent phase then ensues. As TB leads to extensive destruction and fibrosis of organs, thus early diagnosis may prevent function and organ loss. However, nonspecific presentation may result in delayed diagnosis and worsens morbidity (**Table 4.1**).[9]

MICROBIOLOGICAL LABORATORY DIAGNOSIS

The most important step in laboratory diagnosis of UTB is currently based on acid-fast staining and mycobacterial cultures. The gold standard for the TB diagnosis at any site is culture of TB bacilli and in cases of suspected GUTB; it is commonly looked for in the urinary samples. Traditionally, presence of "sterile pyuria" on microscopic examination of urine was considered a classic finding of genitourinary involvement. However, superadded infection with usual coliform bacilli is present in about 30% of the patients. Other findings such as leukocytes in urine, microscopic (50%) or macroscopic (10%), hematuria, and acidic urine are nonspecific and may be absent in 20% of cases.[9]

Microscopy

Urine acid-fast staining (Ziehl-Neelsen) testing, which can be done for GUTB is simple, economical, and rapid but it has low sensitivity and reproducibility. It can identify acid-fast tuberculosis bacilli with a sensitivity of around 40–50%. The poor sensitivity can be explained by sporadic shedding of bacilli in low concentrations and it can be improved by analyzing at least three or preferably five early morning urine samples. Contamination of urine with *Mycobacterium smegmatis* can also give a false positive Ziehl-Neelsen smear result.[9] In addition to being paucibacillary, the nonviscous nature of urine serves as weakening the fixation of bacilli on the smear, thus decreasing the positivity rate of acid-fast bacilli (AFB) smear in urine samples. Another limitation of AFB smear is that nontuberculous mycobacteria like *Mycobacterium smegmatis* can contaminate urine and may lead to false positive result. Despite these disadvantages, AFB smear is still a cost-effective screening tool for EPTB, especially in health settings with high TB burden.[10]

TB Culture

Culture is the gold standard, but has a widely variable sensitivity of 10–80% and can take about 6–8 weeks before the results are obtained, but have the advantage of providing antibiotic sensitivity testing. The urine *Mycobacterium tuberculosis* (MTB) culture test has a higher specificity compared to the urine smear, but as it is time consuming and has long turnaround time, it cannot meet the criteria of point-of-care. Also in comparison with high viscosity of sputum samples, urine samples are watery and more homogeneous, but they require decontamination. The same treatment procedure for both sputum and urine samples appears suitable for sputum, but too rigorous for urine. Hence, one important explanation for low recovery rate by conventional culture methods may be inactivation of a percentage of MTB due to overexposure of tubercle bacilli in the urine samples to the extreme alkaline environment.

MOLECULAR DIAGNOSIS

Nucleic acid amplification (NAA) allows for rapid diagnosis with significantly higher yield even in low bacillary concentrations and can detect mycobacterial DNA in 80.9% patients with suspected GUTB. The sensitivity and specificity of polymerase chain reaction (PCR) on urinary samples range from 94.3 to 95.6% and 85.7 to 94.3%, respectively.[9]

The more recent self-contained cassette based analysis GeneXpert provide results within 2 hours with the advantage of identification of rifampicin (RIF) resistance. The test utilizes five molecular beacons that detect mutations in an 81-bp core region of the *rpoB* gene that are associated with RIF. On the basis of different studies, WHO has recommended GeneXpert to diagnose pulmonary TB and RIF resistant in adults, as well as diagnose EPTB and RIF resistance in adults and children. Unfortunately, given the limited data on the utility in urine samples, these recommendations do not apply on these samples. Few studies have evaluated the performance of the GeneXpert on urine specimen for diagnosis of urinary TB in a country with high TB incidence. One such study showed that compared with L-J culture, AFB microscopy was 40% sensitive while GeneXpert sensitivity was 94%. Also, GeneXpert identified 86% of culture negative UTB cases, yielding a specificity of 86.5%. In clinically diagnosed UTB cases, GeneXpert assay sensitivity was 63% which was significantly higher than L-J culture (45.7%). It shows GeneXpert outperforms AFB smear and solid culture for the detection of MTB in the urine samples, which provides an alternative for the diagnosis of UTB.[10]

In all PCR protocols, possible sources of false positive results are contamination by amplification products aerosolization and false negative results occur due to inhibition by metabolites, drugs, and other body fluid substances. In urine, the most critical inhibitor is urea, which can lead to polymerase degradation in a concentration-dependent manner.[11] While doing PCR, careful controlled protocol avoids both inhibitors as well as contaminants. As Xpert MTB/RIF has inbuilt processing system, it does not face the same problem and is a promising and better diagnostic method for urine than other PCR methods.

Drug resistance information among patients with GUTB is lacking. In this context, none of the Xpert MTB/RIF studies analyzed RIF resistance, possibly because they were done in high-income countries, where multi-drug resistant (MDR) tuberculosis is not usually a concern. One study in China used GenoType® MTBDRplus (Line Probe Assay), which evaluates isoniazid and RIF resistance, in an outpatient setting. They found that one-third of their patients had drug-resistant GUTB, and one-fourth had MDR-GUTB.

Subsequent Xpert MTB/RIF or GenoType® MTBDRplus studies must help characterize drug resistance epidemiology while evaluating the clinical utility of these tests in different MDR prevalence settings.[12]

OTHER DIAGNOSTIC TESTS

Lipoarabinomannan (LAM), a glycolipid component of MTB cell wall, has been used as a promising marker for diagnosing active TB. Several studies found that performance of urinary LAM in unselected TB suspects is unsatisfactory, whereas its diagnostic performance is significantly improved in HIV-infected patients which may be due to the association of renal dysfunction with advanced HIV infection. This test seems suitable for patients who live in settings with high prevalence of HIV. However, with the high frequency of the renal dysfunction due to urinary TB, LAM has the theoretical potential to be an attractive diagnostic option for UTB.[13]

REFERENCES

1. Chauhan LS, Tonsing J. Revised national TB control programme in India. Tuberculosis (Edinb). 2005;85(5-6):271-6.
2. Styblo K. The global aspects of tuberculosis and HIV infection. Bull Int Union Tuberc Lung Dis. 1990;65(1):28-32.
3. Palomino JC. Nonconventional and new methods in the diagnosis of tuberculosis: Feasibility and applicability in the field. Eur Respir J. 2005;26(2): 339-50.
4. Mathew P, Kuo YH, Vazirani B, Eng RH, Weinstein MP. Are three sputum acid-fast bacillus smears necessary for discontinuing tuberculosis isolation? J Clin Microbiol. 2002;40(9):3482-4.
5. Pang Y, Shang Y, Lu J, Liang Q, Dong L, Li Y, et al. Genexpert MTB/RIF assay in the diagnosis of urine tuberculosis from urine specimens. Scientific Reports. 2017;7:6181.
6. Schrader C, Schielke A, Ellerbroek L, Johne R. PCR inhibitors – occurrence, properties and removal. J Appl Microbiol. 2012;113:1014-26.
7. Zheng R, Zhu C, Guo Q, Qin L, Wang J, Lu J, et al. Pyrosequencing for rapid detection of tuberculosis resistance in clinical isolates and sputum samples from re-treatment pulmonary tuberculosis patients. BMC Infect Dis. 2014;14:200.
8. Figueiredo AA, Lucon AM, Junior RF, Srougi M. Epidemiology of urogenital tuberculosis worldwide. Int J Urol. 2008;15(9): 827-32.
9. Yadav S, Singh P, Hemal A, Kumar R. Genital tuberculosis: current status of diagnosis and management. Transl Androl Urol. 2017;6(2):222-33.
10. Pang Y, Shang Y, Lu J, Liang Q, Lingling D, Yunxu L, et al. Genexpert MTB/RIF assay in the diagnosis of urine tuberculosis from urine specimens. Scientific Reports. 2017;7:6181.
11. Schrader C, Schielke A, Ellerbroek L, Johne R. PCR inhibitors–occurrence, properties and removal. J Appl Microbiol. 2012;113:1014-26.
12. Ye Y, Hu X, Shi Y, Zhou J, Zhou Y, Song X, et al. Clinical features and drug resistance profile of urinary tuberculosis in South-Western China: a cross-sectional study. Medicine (Baltimore). 2016;95:e3537.
13. Lawn, SD. Point-of-care detection of lipoarabinomannan (LAM) in urine for diagnosis of HIV-associated tuberculosis: a state of the art review. BMC Infect Dis. 2012;12:103.

CHAPTER 5

Imaging Studies in Genitourinary Tuberculosis

Suleman Merchant, Sujata Patwardhan

This article is based on the original articles of the primary author in reference 1-3. The importance of imaging studies in genitourinary tuberculosis (GUTB) is partly diagnostic and partly to evaluate the extent of the disease involvement, which in turn is used to decide management options. Thus, the imaging plays an integral role in the management of this disease and its follow-up. It is necessary to be familiar with the known diagnostic radiological features as they vary widely and if missed lead to end-stage renal disease (ESRD) in patients. Delay in diagnosis is a grave mistake, which may cost the patient his life. It is usually suggested that radiology cannot be solely used to diagnose the disease either for confirmation or exclusion of patients. Patients with characteristic findings need to be followed up by repeat microbiological tests to prove or exclude the disease.

The changes in the urothelium are best appreciated on the intravenous urography (IVU). It remains the gold standard in spite of other tests like CT, MRI. However, each imaging moderately has something different to offer and hence one or more imaging modalities may be used to get the entire clinical picture or perspective.[1-3]

The plain radiograph:
- Chest X-ray will be positive on 50% of cases with some evidence of past pulmonary disease. Patient may have his old X-ray films of his past diagnosis of pulmonary tuberculosis. Active disease is seen in the chest in 10% of GUTB cases.
- Abdomen plain film may show calcification of abdominal lymph nodes, adrenal glands, prostate vas or seminal vesicles. Evidence of psoas abscess with spine abnormalities, granulomas with calcification in spleen and liver may be seen. Special mention is made about the calcification associated with renal TB. It is considered as the first sign of TB though some consider it to be a sign of advanced or end stage TB kidney; fine calcification is obviously better appreciated on a CT scan.

The pattern of calcification can vary from small areas to complete cast. Initial calcification is faint and punctuate and with time these areas coalesce to form larger areas.

Calcification in the early stage is linear or granular or amorphous and situated within the parenchyma.

Tuberculosis granulomas involving the cortex and medulla are associated with focal globular calcification. Papillary necrosis is associated with triangular ring like calcification within the collecting system. Caseation is associated with homogeneous moderately dense ground glass appearance (putty kidney). Uniform density of 1 cm in diameter calcification is also referred as putty like calcification.[4] Calcific rims outlining the renal lobes is characteristic of TB and is seen in advanced nonfunctioning auto nephrectomy kidneys. This calcification occurs at the junction of necrotic caseous tissue and viable tissue. It is ring shaped as the dilated calyces push the tissue outward.[5]

INTRAVENOUS PYELOGRAM

Intravenous pyelogram (IVP) is considered the best investigation for renal TB because of the depiction of anatomical details. It has been reported that in a series of 45 patients, in 88% of cases diagnosis was possible based on radiology.[4] However, even in active TB, the IVP may be normal in 10–15%. The IVP abnormalities are seen only after the calyx is involved. The initial parenchymal tubercles in the cortex or medulla may not be picked up unless they involve a calyx. The loss of calyceal sharpness can be the first sign along with minimal calyceal dilatation. This is due to mucosal edema.[5] Later on, the calyx wall appear either irregular or ragged, distorted, with moth eaten or feathery appearance, depending upon the disease involvement.[6-9] The author, however, feels that papillary necrosis rather than calyceal erosion is the first sign of TB.

Many a times it is difficult to differentiate papillary necrosis in TB from other causes of papillary necrosis. Papillary erosion in TB is supposed to be more ragged than other causes.[10] At times, an irregular cavity may be seen filled with contrast due to a caseating parenchymal tuberculoma rupturing into adjacent calyx. Elkin feels that this is similar to the picture of papillary necrosis.[5] The papillary necrosis in TB is due to two causes: Ischemia and tissue destruction. The ischemia of the papilla in TB is due to a granuloma involving the papilla or TB endarteritis.

A medullary cavity connected to the pelvicalyceal system (PCS) is a frequent finding on IVP, as reported by Kollens et al.[11] It can involve one or more papilla or bilateral papillae and the cavity can vary in size and outline. Many a times, dilated irregular pools of contrast are seen adjacent to dilated calyces suggestive of a medullary cavity.

Cavitation

Destruction of the parenchyma and adjacent calyx can form a large cavity of necrotic caseous material. Such a cavity may be obstructive or nonobstructive. Contrast material does not enter a cavity which in obstructive on IVU. It is not possible to differentiate a cavity caused by diseased calyx from a cavity caused by granuloma rupturing into a calyx. Nonobstructive cavity is not associated with fibrosis of infundibulum of calyx and can be visualized on retrograde pyelography (RGP). A lipping type of cavity projecting medially has been described.[12] Cavities in renal parenchyma result from enlarging tuberculomas. A kidney destroyed by extensive cavitation is called an ulcerocavernous kidney and is not visualized on IVP. Rupture of cavities into the collecting system lead to further involvement of urothelium and subsequent fibrosis.

Strictures and Scars

Scarring and fibrosis produce more damage than parenchymal tuberculomas. Common sites of fibrosis are infundibulum of calyx, PUJ, and lower ureter. They result in hydrocalyx, regional hydrocalycosis or dilatation of entire PCS.

Strictures occur during period of healing or during the period of treatment with AKT. Strictures of renal pelvis may be due to tuberculous ulceration, however, kinking of the renal pelvis may be due to traction from fibrosed adjacent infundibulum or parenchyma. Such strictures are called "Kirk's Kinks."[13] Scarring of various calyces and a variety of calyceal deformities is unique for tuberculosis, cephalic or upward retraction of the renal pelvis due to stricture of inferior margin of the renal pelvis is described as "Hiked up pelvis."[10]

Obstruction of the kidney due to a pelvic stricture can lead to hydronephrosis and pressure atrophy of renal tissue. However, such hydronephrosis is not smooth and uniform, but have irregular margins and filling defects due to caseous debris.[14] TB can also present as dilated calyces due to pyocalycosis.[1] Stenosis of an infundibulum can lead to nonvisualization of calyx and lack of contrast excretion from involved parenchyma which is described as "phantom calyx."[5] At times, a small part of the infundibulum like a stump or spike may be visualized. Parenchymal scars are seen is 50% of patients and may be either over or in between the calyces.

Late changes in IVP: They are seen as extensive cavities, fibrotic strictures, granulomas causing mass lesions, and extensive calcification.

Limitation of an IVP: A nonvisualized kidney on IVP calls for further investigations. Similarly, a phantom calyx will have to be investigated by a CT or MRI.

Raised creatinine, pregnancy, and allergies to contrast agents would be another cause to use another modality of investigation.

COMPUTED TOMOGRAPHY SCAN

Multidetector computed tomography (MDCT) is useful in diagnosis, in evaluation of the severity of renal involvement,[15] in cases with renal impairment, and in diagnosis of involvement of other organs in abdomen and pelvis. Though CT IVU is replacing conventional IVP due to better details of the anatomy and pathology in multiaxial images, the IVP is still considered supreme for early renal tubercular changes.

The other advantages of the CT include visualization of renal and extra renal spread of disease; it can be used in patients with renal insufficiency.[16,17] It can be done immediately without the need for bowel preparation. MDCT with contrast can evaluate the renal function and degree of obstruction and complications.[18] It is the best modality for a nonvisualized kidney on IVP.

The disadvantages of CT are inability to identify lesions <3 mm and minimal urothelial thickening of a very early change in tuberculosis.

- *Renal parenchymal changes:* Renal granuloma is the first change seen in renal parenchyma in both corticomedullary and nephrographic phases. A granuloma is seen as a solid mass with minimal enhancement after contrast administration along with changes in collecting system.
- *Parenchymal nodules:* Renal TB may present as single or multiple parenchymal nodules with or without collecting system changes. The nodules may vary in size with evidence of peripheral enhancement and hence can be confused as renal neoplasm. Occasionally granulomas can form masses of large size, which are heterogeneous and show areas of calcification. Lu et al.[19] have reported one or more cavities adjacent to calyx with thinning of adjacent cortex as most common finding (68%) in TB.

Computed tomography can identify granulomas containing caseous or calcified material. Active inflammation leading to tissue edema and hypoperfusion may show findings similar to acute bacterial pyelonephritis.

Renal abscesses will be seen as areas of hypodensities (10–40 HU) with mild peripheral enhancement. They may vary in the size and extend into perirenal space. If the abscess is in communication with calyx, it will be seen as irregular pool of contrast material. The abscess may be focal, segmental or involving the entire pole of the kidney. The chronic renal abscess can be confused with cystic renal neoplasm. The clinical history and features of tuberculosis may help in differentiation from a neoplasm, in addition to features such as thickening of Gerota's fascia and perirenal stranding. An aspiration of cavity may be done for culture, sensitivity, and gene expert studies. Fibrosis of parenchyma may be seen located over a deformed calyx or may be unrelated to a calyx. Parenchymal scarring can be seen on CT as an area of global or cortical thinning.

Three imaging patterns have been described by Wang et al. for CT scans in renal TB:
1. Multiple strictures in PC system.
2. Single stricture with other imaging findings.
3. Auto nephrectomy with other imaging findings excluding stricture.

As described earlier, lobar pattern of calcification (lobar caseation) is diagnostic of TB. A combination of abnormalities, which are seen in same patient and recognition of pattern are good pointers toward diagnosis of renal TB.

- *Extrarenal involvement*: CT scan is best diagnostic test for retroperitoneal spread of TB. It helps in identification of involvement of perirenal, pararenal, retroperitoneal and subcutaneous extensions of the renal abscess, adrenal involvement, retroperitoneal fibrosis, psoas abscess, spinal tuberculosis, etc.
- *Fistulas and sinus tract:* As described in the previous section, renal fistulas can involve the kidney and various other organs. CT scan is the most useful modality for diagnosis of fistulas between kidney and alimentary tract. It will depict the intrarenal components, extrarenal inflammation, and the nature of the material/gas present in the PC system.

Renocutaneous fistula can be delineated by injection of contrast material or may be opacified by urine if the kidney is still functioning. The extent of abnormal soft tissue around the sinus tract and extrarenal involvement can be demonstrated. The kidney can communicate with all adjacent structures by a fistula or sinus. They include the skin, bowel, blood lymphatic, liver, pleura, and duodenum. They may be originating either in the parenchyma (renal fistulae) or from the pelvis (pyelo fistulae). Based on the anatomy, fistulae between the duodenum and ascending colon are related to the right kidney and those with the stomach and descending colon are from the left kidney. A rare nephrogluteal fistulae has been described.[20]

Fistulae may also occur between other organs like bowel and bladder.

Adrenal involvement is noted by enlargement in size of adrenal gland central necrosis and calcification. Adrenal atrophy with dense calcification is seen in patients with extensive involvement and Addison's disease.

Features of abdominal tuberculosis such as ascites with septation, omental infiltration, peritoneal thickening, and enlarged lymph node with central necrosis, mesenteric thickening, and bowel wall thickening can be seen on CT scan. Omental calcification along with ascites and necrotic nodes are pathognomonic of abdominal tuberculosis. Secondary renal amyloidosis is known complication of extensive pulmonary tuberculosis and can be diagnosed on CT. TB is the main cause of adrenal insufficiency in Indians.

Calcification: Fine calcification in the parenchyma is a clue to the presence of TB. The types of calcification will vary in size and appearance depending upon the severity of the disease. It may be punctuated, amorphous, and curvilinear surrounded by low attenuated areas of inflammation. The pathognomonic sign of TB is lobar calcification.

Punctuate calcification have been seen in patients with AIDS and atypical mycobacterial (MB) infections in the acute stage of the disease PCS involvement.

Autonephrectomy: Destruction of tissue either due to granulomas or obstruction or both can lead to autonephrectomy. They are of two types viz., the enlarged kidney of the cavernous types with a sac of caseous material or the small shrunken fibrotic, often calcified type of kidney.

Nonvisualization of kidney may be also due to TB arteritis, causing renal vascular hypertension. The disease can involve the intima or subintima with medial hypertrophy and nonfunction. CT or MRI would be the best modality for delineating a nonvisualized kidney on IVP.

Perinephric abscess: The perinephric space can be involved in an abscess either directly from the renal parenchyma, a nearby spine lesion. The spread may be from a psoas abscess or via the blood stream. Rupture of a pyonephrosis or parenchyma abscess is more common route. Though an IVP would suggest a perinephric abscess, the best modality to evaluate an abscess would be a CT/MRI.

Fistulas between PC system and lymphatic system in chyluria can be delineated by CT lymph-angiography.

Chyluria in India in commonly due to TB and filariasis. It will be visualized as pyelosinus and pyelointerstitial back flow. The fistula between the renal fornix and the perirenal lymphatics may be seen. The retroperitoneal lymphatics may be involved with fibrosis. The resultant dilated proximal lymphatics finally find their way to the renal PCS resulting in chyluria.

Strictures: The PCS is mainly involved in GUTB and the pathological features are due to wall ulceration, wall thickening leading to fibrosis and obstruction. Minimal thickening is not well seen on CT scan. However, delayed fibrosis thickening leading to calyectasis is seen well on CT. The most important feature is uneven calyectasis and varying degrees of dilatation at different sites of the kidney. Calyectasis in a nonfunctioning kidney is not revealed in an IVP and is best assessed on a CT scan. Thickening of the renal pelvis and ureter in the early stage and calcification in the late stage can be picked up on CT scan.

As described on the IVU section, the degree of hydronephrosis or calyectasis either focal or generalized will vary upon the site of stricture. The main point to note is the lack of pelvic dilatation in TB.

Fibrosis of the infundibulum, renal pelvis, and ureter can be appreciated on a CT. A very small pelvis or virtually absent pelvis accompanied by calcification is described as daisy flower appearance.

Calyces that contain urine have a HU of 0–10, those with debris have HU of 10–30, those having putty material have HU of 50–120, and calcification have a HU of 120 HU or more.

Lobar caseation is a characteristic of renal TB. The calyces are dilated, crowded or assimilated into the caseous renal parenchyma. They do not communicate with each other. Unequal calyectasis with urothelial thickening in the absence of obstructive calculi should point toward TB.

Many authors have stated that a combination of various radiological abnormalities in the same renal unit is considered to be suggestive of renal TB.

Kenny[21] has stated that a combination of pelvic infundibular strictures, papillary necrosis, and cortical low attenuating masses with calcification is highly suggestive of TB.

MAGNETIC RESONANCE IMAGING

Magnetic resonance imaging (MRI) is particularly useful in pregnant and pediatric cases, when iodinated contrast cannot be administered. Noncontrast MRI and magnetic resonance urography (MRU) can be utilized to demonstrate renal tuberculosis. MRI provides better delineation of morphological details of the kidney and the ureters. Since MRU is useful for evaluation of the ureters in dilated, obstructed systems with impaired renal functions. Very few articles are available regarding use of MRI for diagnosis of TB. Though, the superior contrast resolution of MRI is ideal for this disease. MRI may be useful when CT and ultrasonography (USG) are equivocal.

Renal Parenchyma

Renal parenchymal involvement is visualized as local hypoperfusion due to local tissue edema and vasoconstriction. Asymmetrical perinephric fat stranding, thickening of Gerota's fascia and loss of interface between renal parenchyma, and the infections focus may be clues to indicate that local infection is due to TB.

T1-weighted (T1W) images will very well show the hypoperfused areas along with focal calyectasis and urothelial thickening. MRI would be the best method to demonstrate present or absence of enhancement within the renal mass. However, it would be necessary to coregister the unenhanced and contrast enhanced images and perform the MRI sequences during the end expiratory breath holding.

Granulomas

Small nodules appear as hypointense areas both in T1W and T2-weighted (T2W) images; large nodules appear as central hyperintense areas in T2W images. Necrotic debris and caseation cause heterogeneous hypo or isointense signals on T2W images. At time, caseation may appear as hyperintense on T2W image. Still larger granulomas may show a thick irregular hypointense collection with debris, fluid level. The parenchymal granuloma/nodule may be associated with PC system involvement. A larger nodule may mimic a neoplasm.

Magnetic resonance imaging will help in differentiation of macronodular TB and malignancy. Apparent diffusion coefficient is decreased in renal fibrosis and is associated with increase in number of fibroblast and has been suggested as a server to noninvasive biomarker of renal fibrosis. Experimental animal studies have used this component of diffusion weighted MRI to evaluate fibrosis. It may be utilized in the follow-up of the disease.[22] Renal anisotropy is used to reflect the nephron architecture and a possible biomarker in the future. MRI elastography has been useful in the evaluation of renal tuberculosis and the following after treatment.

Collecting Systems

Diffusion-weighted imaging (DWI) can be used to detect changes in the collecting system, and the presence of multifocal stricture an uneven/unequal calyectasis. Small renal pelvis associated with scarring and urothelial thickening can be diagnostic of tuberculosis.

Magnetic resonance urography is used for the evaluation of calyectasis and hydronephrosis in nonfunctioning kidney. DWI can be used to differentiate between hydronephrosis and pyonephrosis; however, this finding cannot be specific for tuberculosis. In general, DWI can detect and characterize focal lesions, diffuse parenchymal disease multiloculated cysts in which other techniques may be suboptimal.

MAGNETIC RESONANCE ANGIOGRAPHY

Renal MR angiography can be utilized when renovascular hypertension is suspected due to TB. Pruning of the peripheral vessels with hypovascular masses and reduced blood flow, narrowing of the intrarenal vessels, can be diagnosed on angiography. It may be used in the planning of partial nephrectomy, if required.

TUBERCULOSIS IN TRANSPLANTED KIDNEY

It can occur due to immunocompromised state. Pulmonary followed by GUTB within a period of 6–7 months can be seen in patients undergoing transplant.[23] It can also be due to pre-existing TB in donor kidney. TB in renal transplant has been reported in 17.86% of cases.[24] Factors associated with increased risk of TB in transplant kidney are cyclosporin, DM2, post-transplant rejection, and chronic liver disease.[25] Imaging findings are nonspecific. IVP is relatively inferior modality to evaluate the PC system in the transplanted kidney.[23] Corticosteroid treatment for transplant recipients account for lack of features of TB, usually seen on an IVU. Imaging, thus, in a transplant patient may not be able to diagnose the disease as early than in an index GUTB patient, other test like microbiology of urine will be necessary.

REFERENCES

1. Merchant SA. Tuberculosis of the genitourinary system. Indian J Radiol Imaging. 1993;3:253-74.
2. Merchant S, Bharati A, Merchant N. Tuberculosis of the genitourinary system-Urinary tract tuberculosis: Renal tuberculosis-Part I. Indian J Radiol Imaging 2013;23:46-63
3. Merchant S, Bharati A, Merchant N. Tuberculosis of the genitourinary system-Urinary tract tuberculosis: Renal tuberculosis-Part II. Indian J Radiol Imaging 2013;23:64-77
4. Premkumar A, Lattimer J, Newhouse JH. CT and sonography of advanced urinary tract tuberculosis. AJR Am J Roentgenol. 1987;148:65-9.
5. Elkin M. Urogenital tuberculosis. In: Pollack HM, (Ed). Clinical Urography. Philadelphia: WB Saunders; 1990. pp. 1020-52.
6. Tonkin AK, Witten DM. Genitourinary tuberculosis. Semin Roentgenol. 1979;14:305-18.
7. Brasch WF. Roentgenographic diagnosis in renal tuberculosis. Surg Gynecol Obst. 1919;28:555-61.
8. Taylor H. Renal tuberculosis pathogenesis and Roentgen findings. AJR Am J Roentgenol. 1939;42:700-8.
9. Benjamin JA, Taylor HB. Renal tuberculosis and tuberculous perinephric abscess. J Urol. 1945;53:265-8.
10. Becker JA. Renal tuberculosis. Urol Radiol. 1988;10:25-30.
11. Kollins SA, Hartman GW, Carr DT, Segura JW, Hattery RR. Roentgenographic findings in urinary tract tuberculosis. A 10 year review. Am J Roentgenol Radium Ther Nucl Med. 1974;121:487-99.
12. Frimann-Dahl J. Radiological investigations of urogenital tuberculosis. Urol Int. 1955;1:396-426.
13. Barrie HJ, Kerr WK, Gale GL. The incidence and pathogenesis of tuberculous strictures of the renal pyelus. J Urol. 1967;98:584-9.
14. Burrill J, Williams CJ, Bain G, Conder G, Hine AL, Misra RR. Tuberculosis: A radiologic review. Radiographics. 2007;27:1255-73.
15. Qunibi WY, al-Sibai MB, Taher S, et al. Mycobacterial infection after renal transplantation–Report of 14 cases and review of the literature. Q J Med. 1990;77:1039-60.
16. Rose AG. Diseases of medium-sized arteries, including hypertension. In: Silver MD (Ed). Cardiovascular Pathology, 1st edition. New York: Churchill Livingstone Inc; 1983. pp. 739-76.
17. Rui X, Li XD, Cai S, Chen G, Cai B. Ultrasonographic diagnosis and typing of renal tuberculosis. Int J Urol. 2008;15:135-9.

18. Browne RF, Zwirewich C, Torreggiani WC. Imaging of urinary tract infection in the adult. Eur Radiol. 2004;14:E168-83.
19. Lu P, Li C, Zhou X. Significance of the CT scan in renal tuberculosis. Zhonghua Jie He He Hu Xi Za Zhi. 2001;24:407-9.
20. Hanchanale V, Rao A, Motiwala H. Renogluteal fistula: An unusual complication of genitourinary tuberculosis. Indian J Urol. 2006;22:270-1.
21. Kenney PJ. Imaging of chronic renal infections. AJR Am J Roentgenol. 1990;155:485-94.
22. Fan ZM, Zeng QY, Huo JW, et al. Macronodular multiorgans tuberculoma: CT and MR appearances. J Gastroenterol. 1998;33:285-8.
23. Dowdy L, Ramgopal M, Hoffman T, et al. Genitourinary tuberculosis after renal transplantation: Report of 3 cases and review. Clin Infect Dis. 2001;32:662-6.
24. Zhang XF, Lv Y, Xue WJ, et al. Mycobacterium tuberculosis infection in solid organ transplant recipients: Experience from a single centre in China. Transplant Proc. 2008;40:1382-5.
25. Mercadal L, Foltz V, Isnard-Bagnis C, Ourahma S, Deray G. Tuberculosis after conversion from azathioprine to mycophenolate mofetil in a long-term renal transplant recipient. Transplant Proc. 2005;37:4241-3.

CHAPTER 6

Sonographic Features of Urinary Tuberculosis

S Boopathy Vijayaraghavan

In case of urinary tuberculosis, several lesions can be viewed on sonography and the features are well seen on high-resolution ultrasonography (HRUS) using the high-frequency probe from 5 to 12 MHz utilizing recent techniques like compound imaging and harmonics. The sonographic features of urinary tuberculosis reveal its pathological process. The salient features of urinary tuberculosis on sonography are involvement of multiple areas of the urinary tract and visualization of different stages of the disease in the same patient In the renal parenchyma, the coalescent granulomas are visible as masses of different sizes as well as varied echogenicity; usually, these are visible as masses of mixed echogenicity, which can be with or without necrotic areas of caseation (**Figs. 6.1A and B and 6.2**). Few granulomas may reveal punctate calcifications (**Figs. 6.3A and B**). Both cavitation as well as caseation in the granuloma can be viewed as parenchymal cavities of different sizes (**Figs. 6.4 and 6.5**), and few of them are very close to the calyces distorting them (**Fig. 6.4**). Upon rupturing of the cavity into the calyx, the communication is shown as an anechoic tract, between the parenchymal cavity and the calyx (**Fig. 6.6**). In case

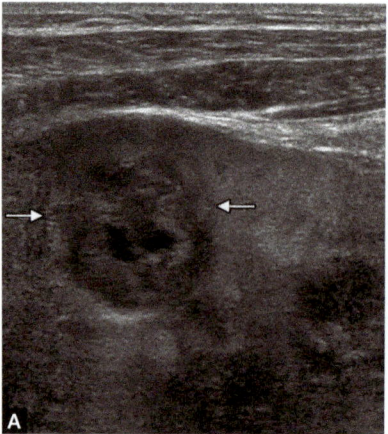 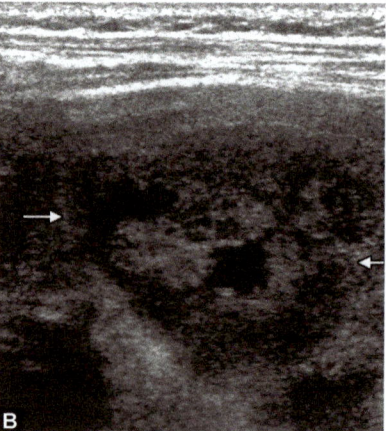

FIGS. 6.1A AND B: High-resolution ultrasonography (HRUS) images of the kidney showing (A) parenchymal mass (arrows) of mixed echogenicity and (B) a mass (arrows) with an area of caseation and cavitation.

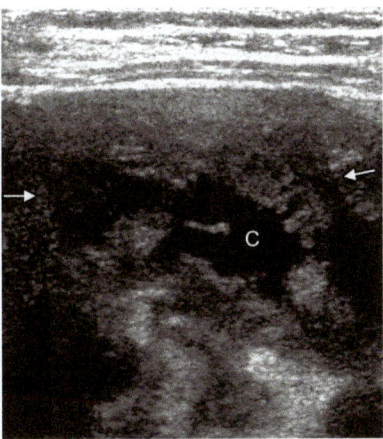

FIG. 6.2: High-resolution ultrasonography (HRUS) images of the kidney showing a large irregular parenchymal cavity (C) within an echopoor mass (arrows).

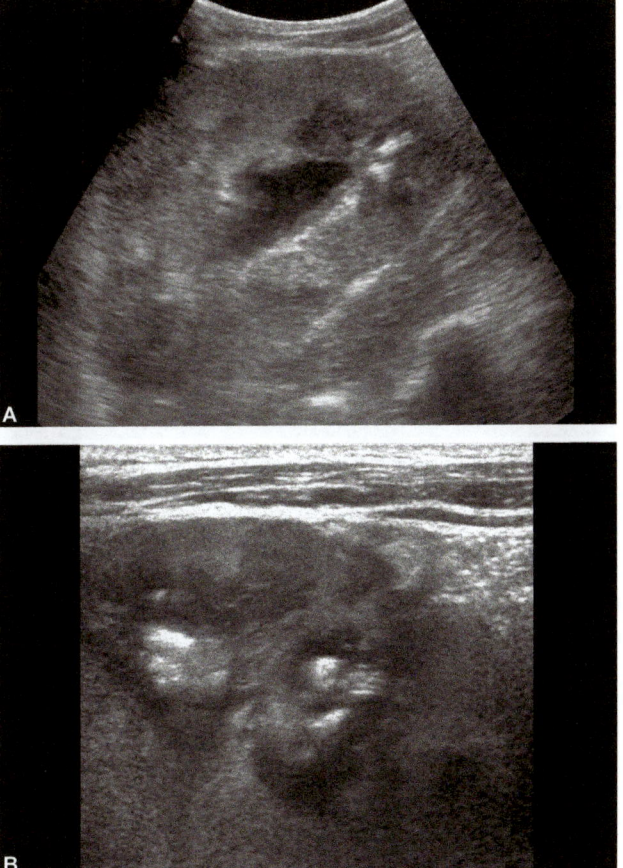

FIGS. 6.3A AND B: (A) Sagittal scan and (B) High-resolution ultrasonography (HRUS) image of the kidney showing parenchymal masses with calcifications in them.

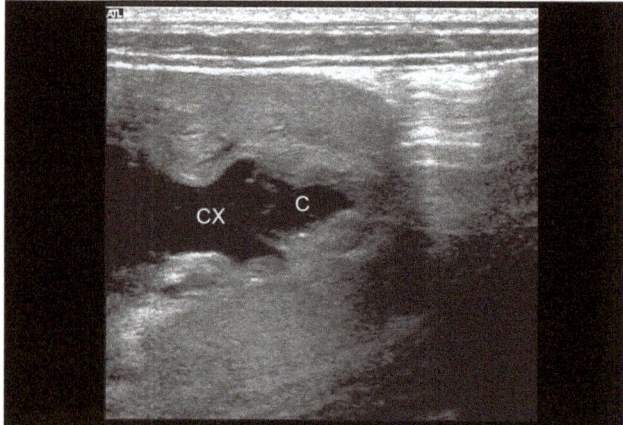

FIG. 6.4: High-resolution ultrasonography (HRUS) image of the kidney showing the lower pole calyx (CX) and a large medullary cavity (C) distorting the calyx.

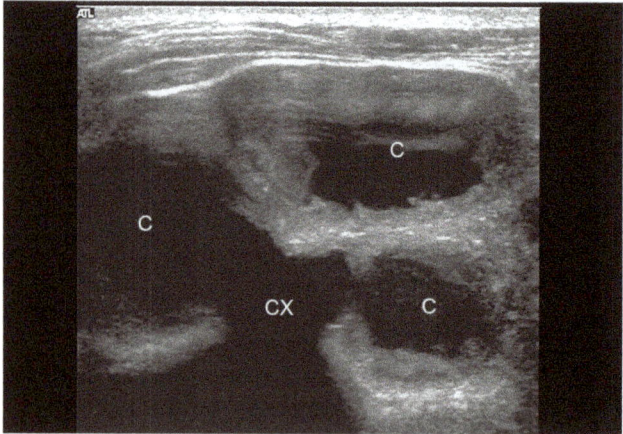

FIG. 6.5: High-resolution ultrasonography (HRUS) image of the kidney showing a sloughed necrosed papilla (P) in the calyx.

of marked destruction of the papilla, the resulting cavity is visible in continuity with the calyx having a broad communication. Sloughed necrosed papilla in the cavity is seen very rarely (**Fig. 6.5**). Quite often, there is an extension of the cavity externally, which ruptures into perinephric space, and is shown as a perinephric abscess in the sonographic study (**Fig. 6.7A**). This abscess can further extend into the abdominal wall (**Fig. 6.7B**) and rupture externally that leads to formation of the nephrocutaneous fistula, which is seen as a hypoechoic tract (**Fig. 6.7C**) from perinephric space to skin.[1]

The involvement of collecting system is visible as irregular mucosal thickening of varied degree in the calyces and the pelvis (**Figs. 6.8 to 6.10**), owing to the inflammation, granulomas, caseation, and ulceration of the urothelium. At the site of anatomic narrowing, lesions are very common or frequent. For instance, at the infundibula of the calyces, the

Sonographic Features of Urinary Tuberculosis 63

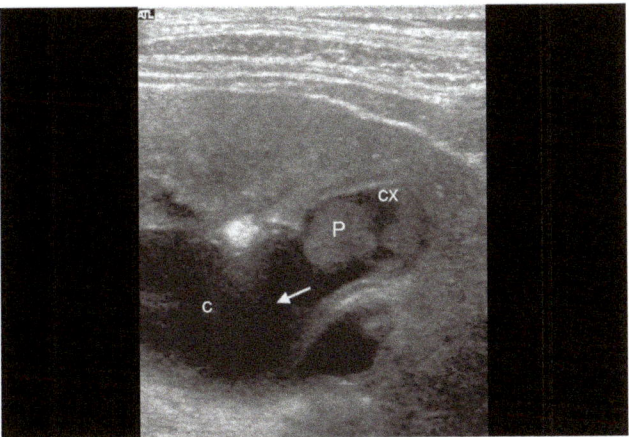

FIG. 6.6: High-resolution ultrasonography (HRUS) images of the kidney showing an irregular medullary cavity (c) communicating by a sonolucent tract (arrow) with the calyx.

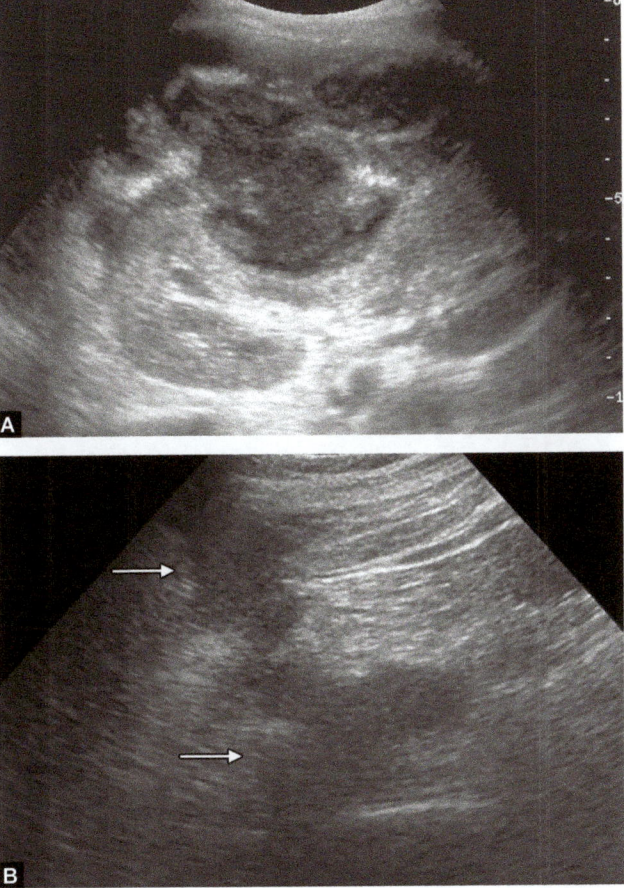

FIGS. 6.7A TO C: *Continued...*

Continued...

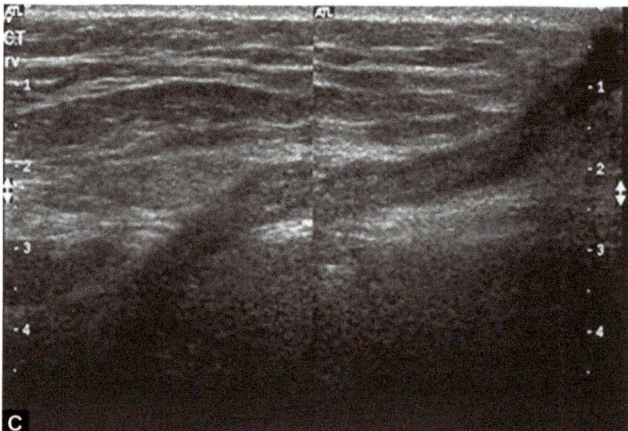

FIGS. 6.7A TO C: (A) Coronal scan of the kidney showing renal and perinephric abscess. (B) Scan of the left flank showing extension of a tuberculous perinephric abscess into the posterior abdominal wall (arrows). (C) Scan of the left flank shows an echopoor tract extending to the perinephric space from the skin.

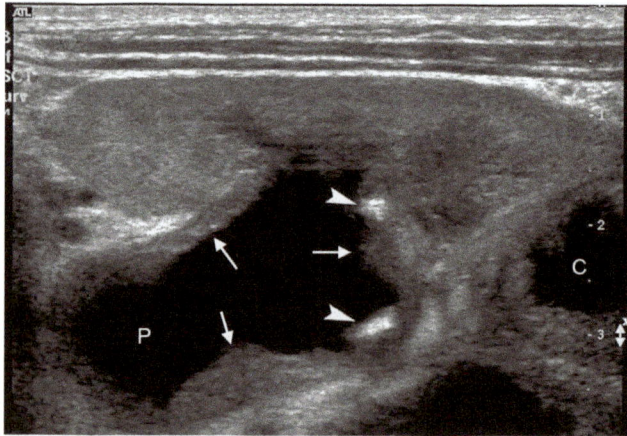

FIG. 6.8: High-resolution ultrasonography (HRUS) image of transverse scan of the kidney showing mucosal thickening (arrows) of calyces and pelvis (P). There are calcifications of wall of calyx and pelvis (arrow heads). A parenchymal cavity (C) is also seen.

pelviureteric junction, and the ureterovesical junction. There is mucosal thickening and narrowing of the lumen and proximal dilatation in case of lesions in the ureter (**Fig. 6.11**). In case lesions are present on multiple sites in the ureter, the lumen of the ureter represents a beaded appearance due to alternate areas of the mucosal thickening (**Fig. 6.12**) with intervening dilatation.

The main characteristic of tuberculosis is that both the destructive as well as the healing features due to fibrosis and calcification can be seen alongside in sonography. There are parenchymal scars with or without calcification (**Fig. 6.13**). Healing of a parenchymal cavity may lead to formation of tiny parenchymal cyst with milk of calcium (**Fig. 6.14**). In the collecting system, the sites of anatomic narrowing are usually the sites for fibrous

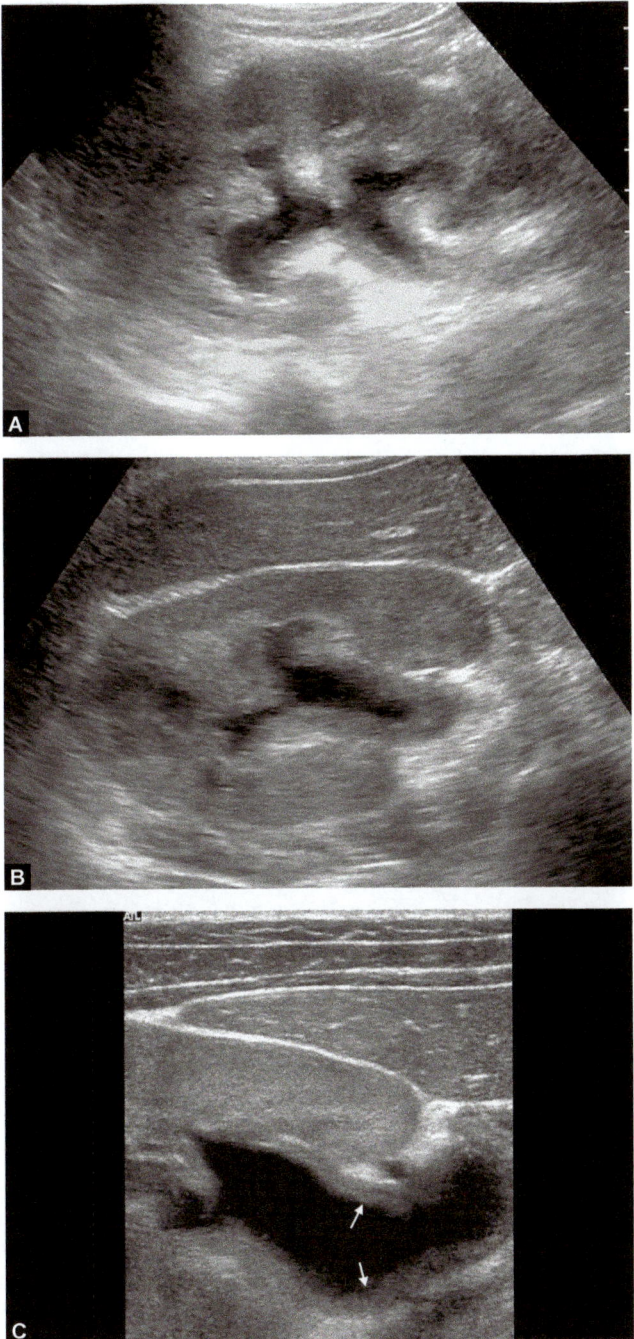

FIGS. 6.9A TO C: (A) Coronal and (B) transverse scans of the kidney showing (C) mucosal thickening in the calyces and pelvis. High-resolution ultrasonography (HRUS) image of the same patient.

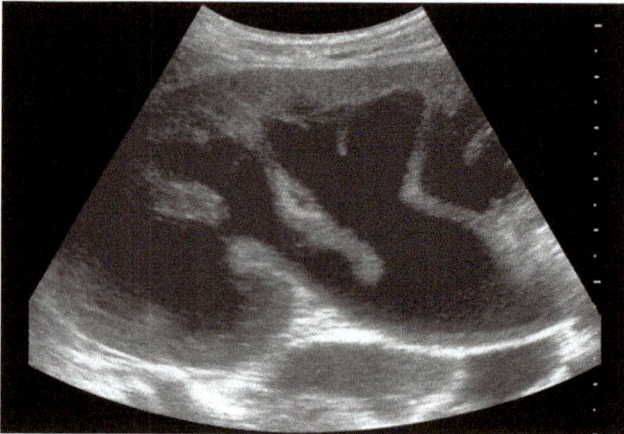

FIG. 6.10: Coronal scan showing hydronephrosis due to stenosis of pelviureteric junction. A Mucosal thickening of calyces and pelvis is also seen.

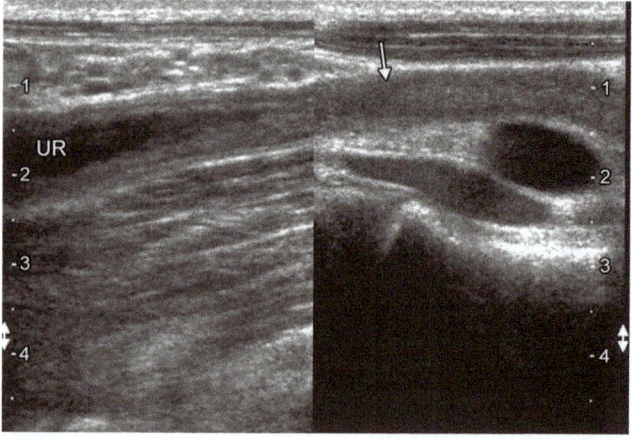

FIG. 6.11: High-resolution ultrasonography (HRUS) image of the midureter showing marked mucosal thickening (arrow) of the ureter obliterating the lumen with dilated proximal ureter (UR).

scarring. Focal caliectasis is caused by the narrowing of the infundibulum of the calyx (**Figs. 6.15A and B**). In case of presence of a stricture in the pelvis, the characteristic feature seen is uneven or asymmetric caliectasis, which means that some calyces are grossly dilated, some are slightly dilated, and some are not dilated (**Fig. 6.16**). In case of involvement of all the calyces, there occurs asymmetric or symmetric dilatation of all the calyces without renal pelvis dilatation (**Fig. 6.17**). Fibrosis of the involved parenchyma, the infundibulum, and the pelvis causes some part of the kidney to be retracted and the remaining part of the kidney to be dilated which leads to kinking and distortion of the renal pelvis, called Kerr's kink (**Figs. 6.18A and B**). Hydronephrosis (**Fig. 6.10**) or pyonephrosis can be caused due to fibrotic healing of the pelviureteric junction (**Fig. 6.19**). Fibrosis in the ureter leads to single or multiple strictures with hydronephrosis (**Fig. 6.20**). It may also

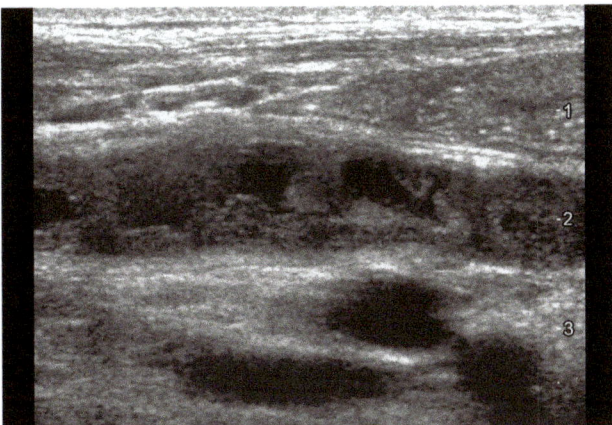

FIG. 6.12: High-resolution ultrasonography (HRUS) image of the midureter showing the beaded appearance due to multiple segments of marked mucosal thickening.

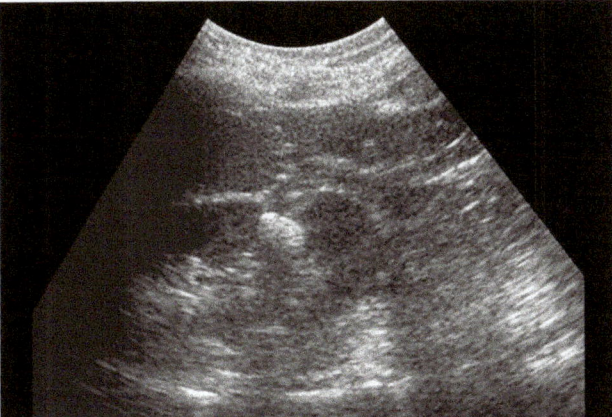

FIG. 6.13: Coronal scan of the kidney showing a parenchymal scar with a mass of calcification deep to it.

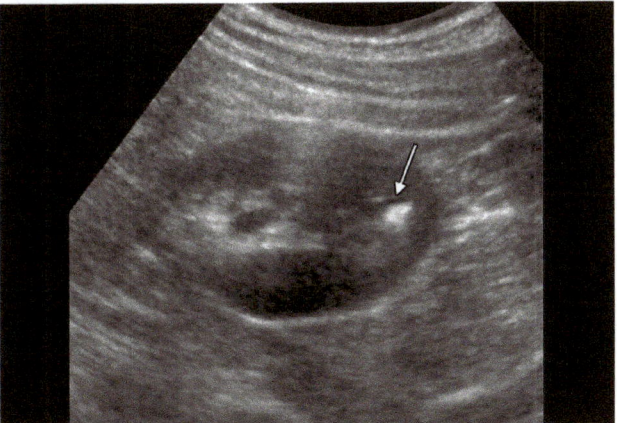

FIG. 6.14: Transverse scan of the upper pole of the left kidney shows a small parenchymal cyst with milk of calcium (arrow) due to the healing of a parenchymal cavity.

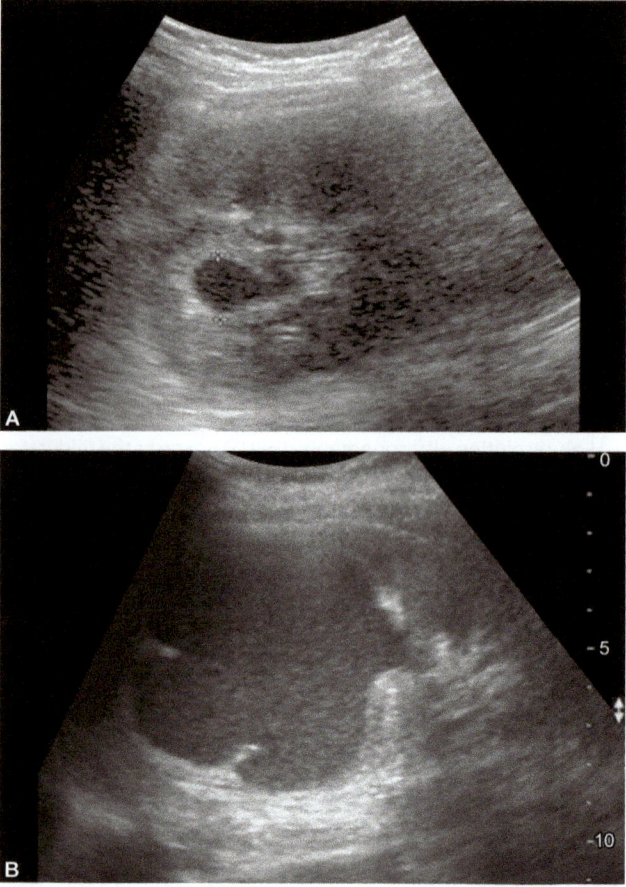

FIGS. 6.15A AND B: (A) Coronal scan of upper pole of left kidney shows a focal caliectasis of a minor calyx due to stenosis of its infundibulum. (B) Coronal scan of right kidney showing major caliectasis due to fibrosis of the infundibulum of upper major calyx.

lead to straight, rigid tube with a patulous ureteric orifice and vesicoureteric reflux in the lower ureter (**Figs. 6.21A and B**). In the urinary bladder, mucosal tubercles coalesce and produce ulceration and edema; the common sites of involvement are around the ureteric orifices (**Figs. 6.22A and B**). Ureteral obstruction can be caused by edema in trigonal mucosa (**Fig. 6.21A**). Greater involvement of the bladder mucosa leads to potentially reversible decrease in capacity of the bladder, most likely owing to the spasm (**Fig. 6.23**). The progression of the inflammation involves the muscular layer and mural fibrosis and results in significant thickening of the wall of the bladder. This leads to irreversible contraction of urinary bladder resulting in a thimble bladder (**Fig. 6.24**). Fibrosis in the trigone region can cause gaping in ureteric orifice and may also cause vesicoureteric reflux (**Fig. 6.21B**). The process of healing includes calcification of the lesions. It can either be seen as clumps of punctate calcification (**Figs. 6.3A and B**) or a lobar type of calcification deep to a scar in the renal parenchyma (**Fig. 6.13**). If the dystrophic calcifications are diffuse and uniform, they are called putty-like calcification, a hallmark of renal tuberculosis. Whereas, in case of

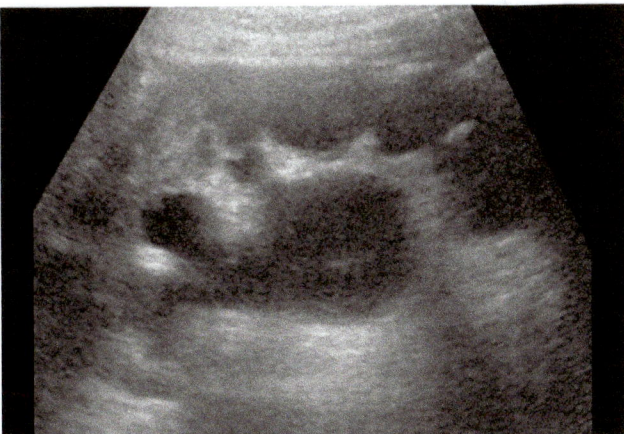

FIG. 6.16: Coronal scan showing asymmetric caliectasis—marked dilatation of lower calyces, moderate dilatation of upper calyx, and normal middle calyx.

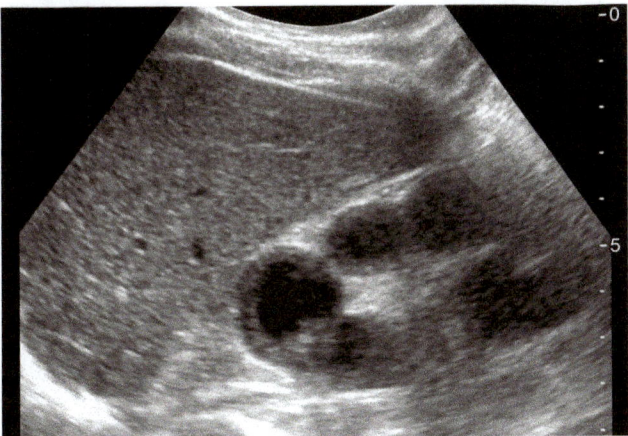

FIG. 6.17: Coronal scan of the kidney showing dilatation of all the calyces without renal pelvis dilatation due to pelvic stricture.

extensive calcification, the appearance is called "putty kidney" (**Fig. 6.25**). In the collecting system, when focal, it can be viewed as speckled or curvilinear calcifications in the wall of the calyx (**Fig. 6. 8**), pelvis (**Fig. 6.26**), and the ureter. In case of widespread dystrophic calcification of the hydronephrotic nonfunctioning kidney, a cast of kidney is formed ,which is also called as an autonephrectomy (**Fig. 6.27**).

DIFFERENTIAL DIAGNOSIS

Hence, it can be said that sonography can be used for visualizing a myriad of conditions caused due to urinary tuberculosis and each of these can be resultant of various other disease processes, for instance due to papillary necrosis of different forms, malignant lesions in kidney and the collecting system, and also bacterial cystitis. The chief characteristic feature of urinary tuberculosis on sonography is presence of lesions in

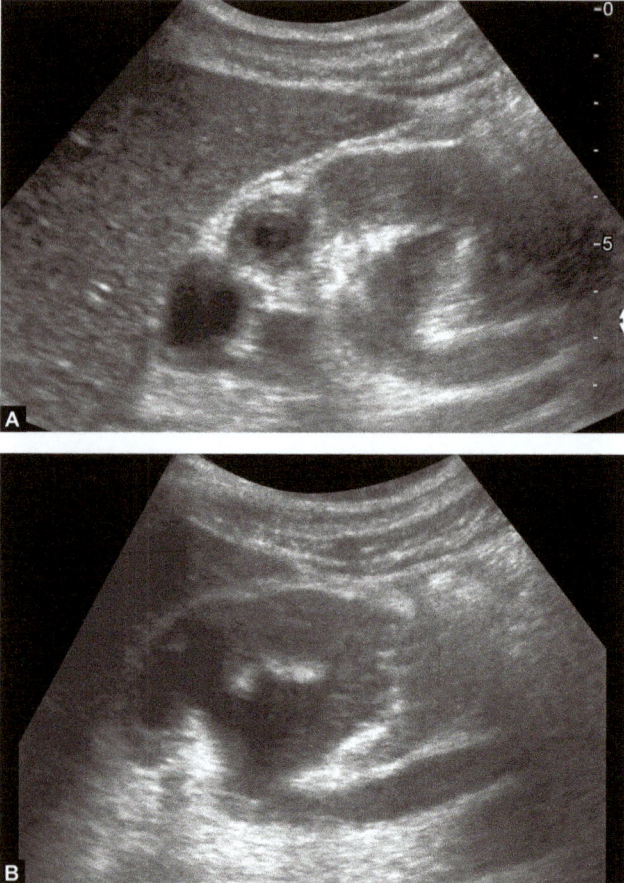

FIGS. 6.18A AND B: (A) Coronal scan of the kidney showing multiple parenchymal cavities in the upper pole. (B) On healing with fibrosis, it has resulted in the distortion and kinking of the renal pelvis.

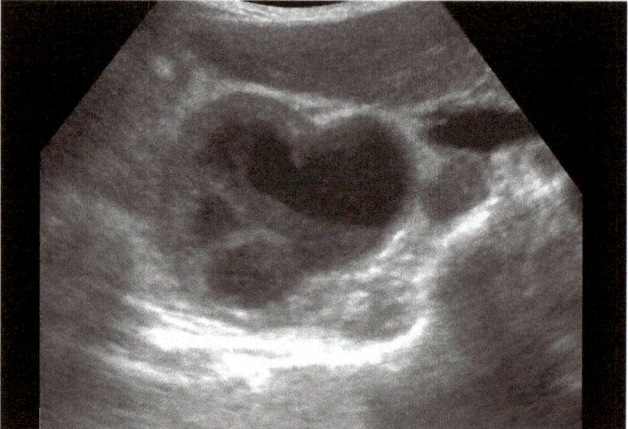

FIG. 6.19: Transverse scan of the kidney showing pyonephrosis with debris in dilated calyces.

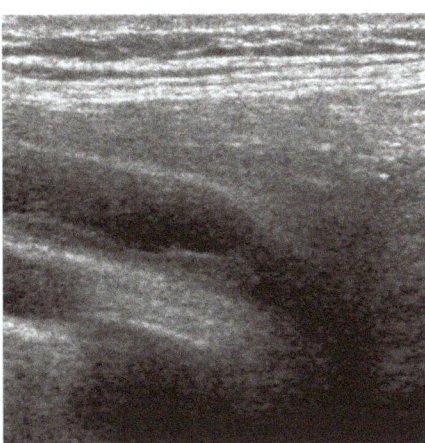

FIG. 6.20: Oblique scan of midureter showing stricture at the level of pelvic brim and dilated proximal ureter.

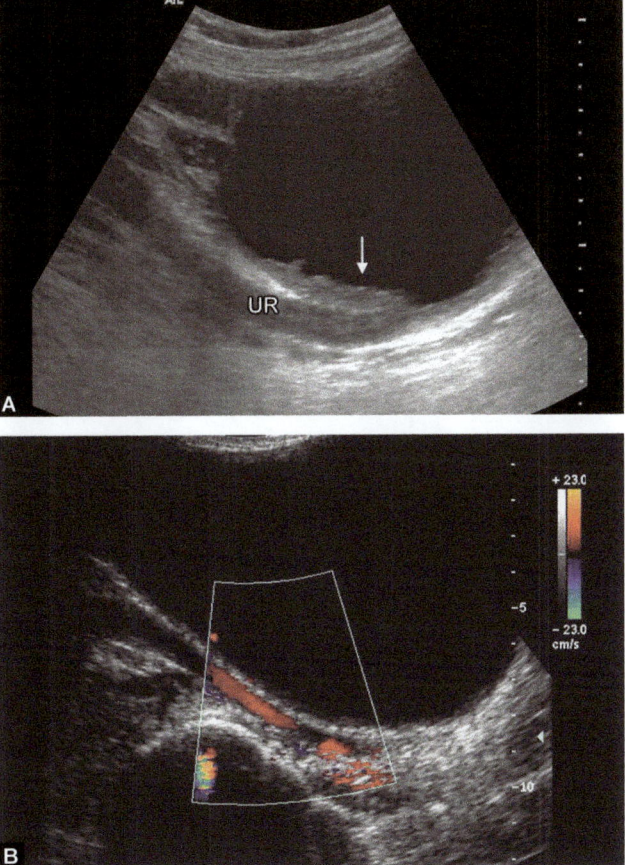

FIGS. 6.21A AND B: (A) Oblique scan of urinary bladder and ureter showing mucosal thickening of trigone area (arrow) and distal ureter (UR) with dilated proximal ureter. (B) Color Doppler image of the ureter showing the vesicoureteric reflux due to healing and fibrosis.

72 Genitourinary Tuberculosis

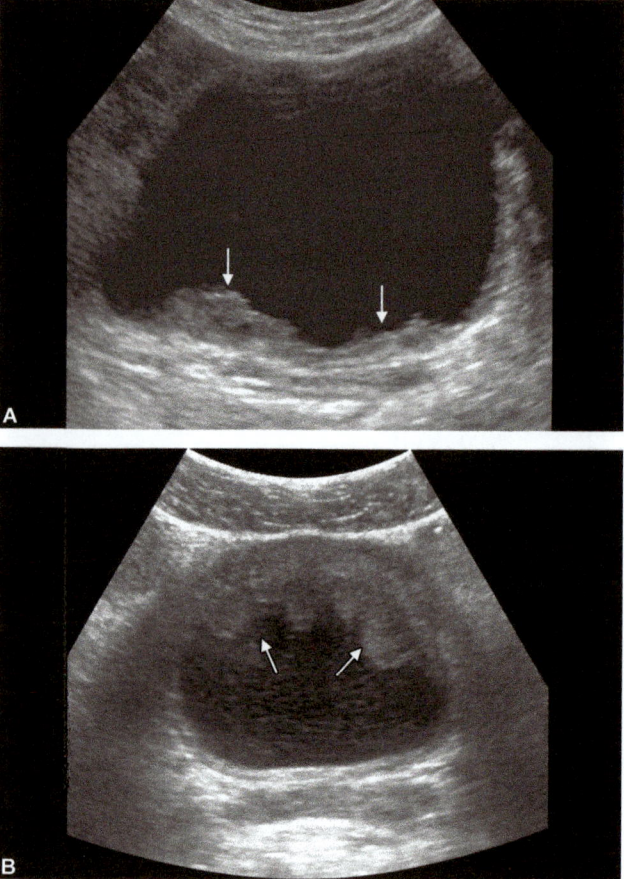

FIGS. 6.22A AND B: Transverse scan of urinary bladder showing focal irregular mucosal thickening (arrows) in region of (A) trigone and (B) anterior wall.

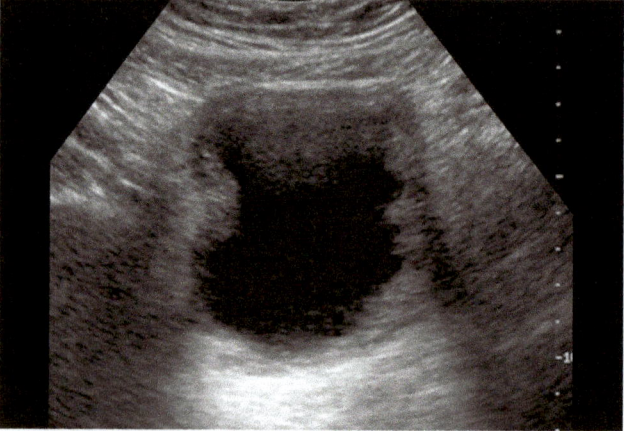

FIG. 6.23: Marked mucosal thickening of most of the urinary bladder resulting in a reversible decrease in capacity.

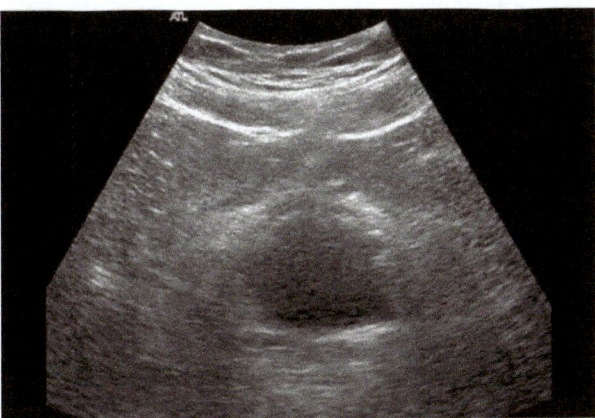

FIG. 6.24: Fibrosis of the walls of the urinary bladder resulting in an irreversible thick-walled small volume urinary bladder—thimble bladder.

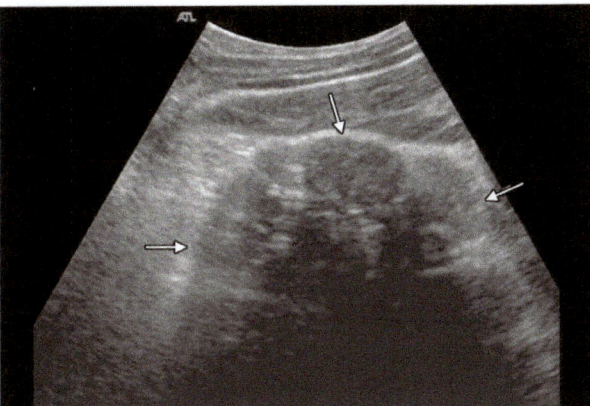

FIG. 6.25: Coronal scan of the renal area showing the extensive calcification of the kidney (arrows) with shadowing characteristic of a "putty kidney."

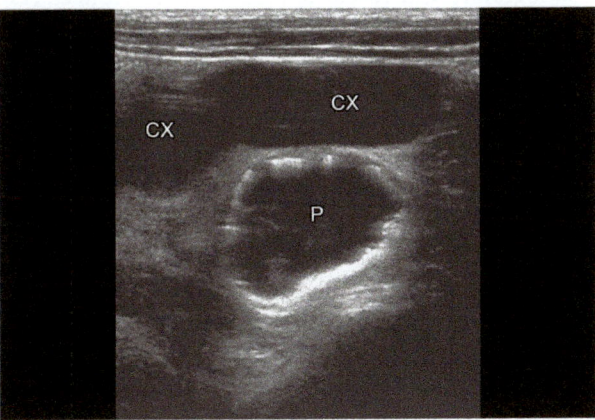

(CX: calyx)

FIG. 6.26: Transverse scan of a grossly hydronephrotic kidney showing extensive calcification of wall of renal pelvis (P).

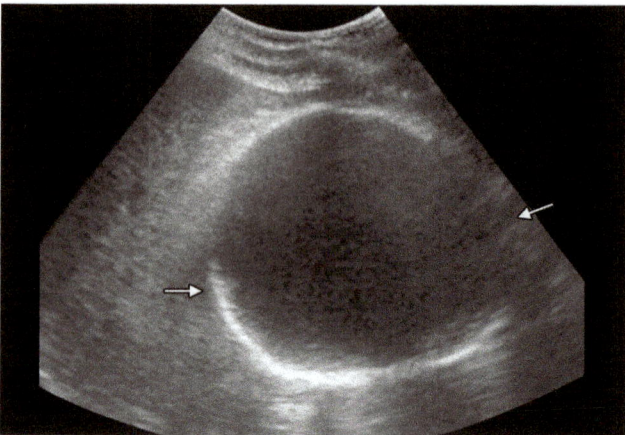

FIG. 6.27: Coronal scan of the renal area showing the calcified walls of the hydronephrotic kidney (arrows)—autonephrectomy.

multiple areas in urinary tract, and visualization of different stages of the disease in the same patient along with chronic nature of the symptoms.

MALE GENITAL TRACT

Prostate

In prostate gland, sonography is carried through the transrectal route. In most of the TB patients, sonography does not reveal any lesions in the prostate. In some cases, focal areas of decreased echogenicity may be visible (**Fig. 6.28**). There may be dystrophic calcifications (**Fig. 6.29**). In prostate, an abscess may rarely be present with or without periprostatic collection (**Figs. 6.30A and B**); it can mimic a pyogenic abscess, especially in immunocompromised state. In rarity, a fistulous tract to perineum or an air-filled tract extending from prostate to the anal canal may be seen which is indicative of an anourethral fistula (**Figs. 6.31A to C**). In patients who present with infertility, because of ejaculatory duct obstruction, sonography will reveal dilated seminal vesicles (**Figs. 6.32A and B**) in association to dilated tubules in the epididymis (**Figs. 6.33A and B**). There may be a possibility of ectasia of rete testis (**Fig. 6.34**) and epididymal cysts (**Fig. 6.35**). Prostatic lesions have a nonspecific appearance and can mimic appearances of malignancy or any other nonspecific infection. In case the symptoms are chronic, or in presence of additional features of urinary tuberculosis, biopsy is unnecessary. In other cases, a guided biopsy or aspiration is done for ruling out tuberculosis. In the chronic type of lesions such as fibrosis and calcifications, to prove the infection is highly impossible and not mandatory, because the treatment is directed toward relieving the major symptoms such as obstruction or correcting the fistula instead of tuberculosis.

Epididymal and Testicular Tuberculosis

In tuberculosis patients, sonography of scrotum reveals significant heterogeneity in relation to pathologic components like caseous necrosis, fibrosis, granulomas, and calcifications. Tuberculous epididymitis presents as diffusely enlarged heterogeneously hypoechoic epididymis (**Figs. 36A and B**) and may be presence of nodular heterogeneous hypoechoic

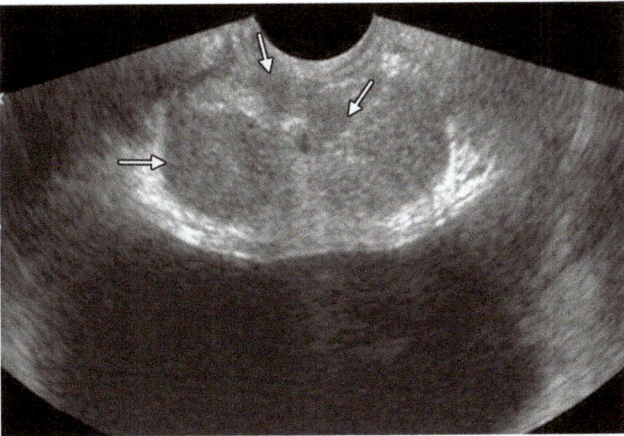

FIG. 6.28: Transrectal ultrasound image shows ill-defined echopoor areas in prostate (arrows).

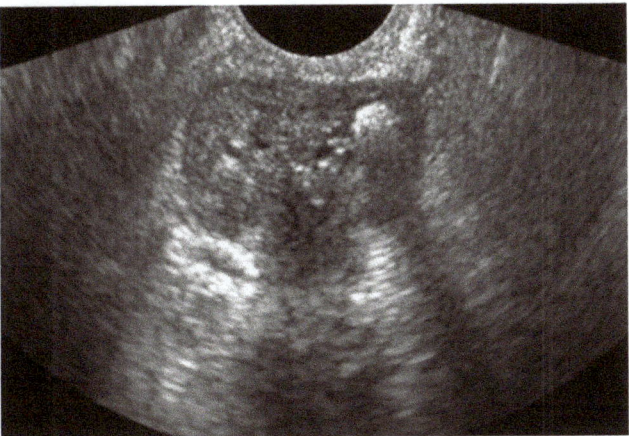

FIG. 6.29: Healing of granulomas results in dystrophic calcifications in the prostate.

lesions in the epididymis (**Figs. 37A and B**). The Color Doppler study can reveal few vessels in the periphery of epididymis without the flow in the focal lesions (**Fig. 6.36B**). The epididymis is rarely diffusely enlarged and homogeneously hypoechoic (**Fig. 6.38**). When the infection is aggressive, an abscess may mimic a pyogenic infection (**Figs. 6.39A and B**). There may be an outspread of the abscess into the wall of the scrotum (**Fig. 6.40**). In case of scrotal sinus, there is a possibility of an echopoor or fluid-filled tract, mostly tail, which extends from the epididymis, into the wall of the scrotum and up to the skin (**Fig. 6.41**). Thickening of the scrotum wall; calcification of epididymis (**Fig. 6.42**); tunica vaginalis (**Fig. 6.43**); and hydrocele (**Fig. 6.44**) can also be present. In case of tuberculous orchitis, common features or appearances include the following:
- Diffused enlargement of testis with multiple small, homogeneous or heterogeneous hypoechoic nodules (**Fig. 6.44**).
- Blurring of the separation between the testis and epididymis (**Fig. 6.45**).

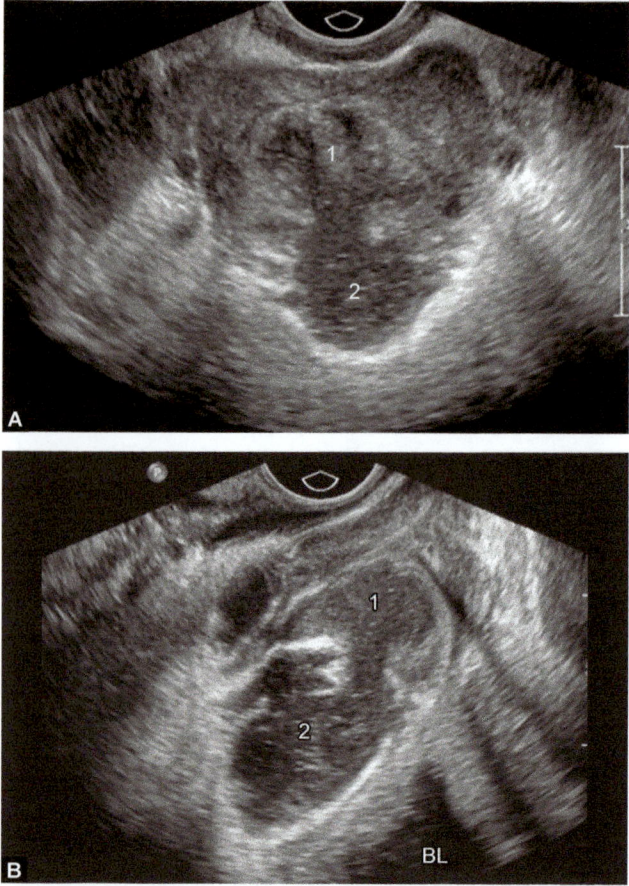

FIGS. 6.30A AND B: (A) Axial and (B) longitudinal scans of the prostate showing an abscess (1) which extends outside the gland (2).

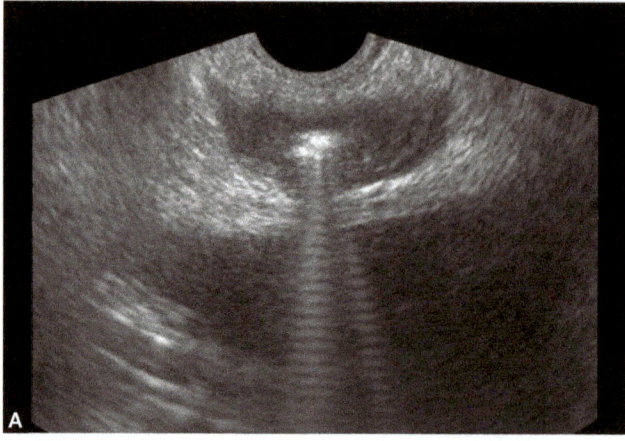

FIGS. 6.31A TO C:

Continued...

Continued...

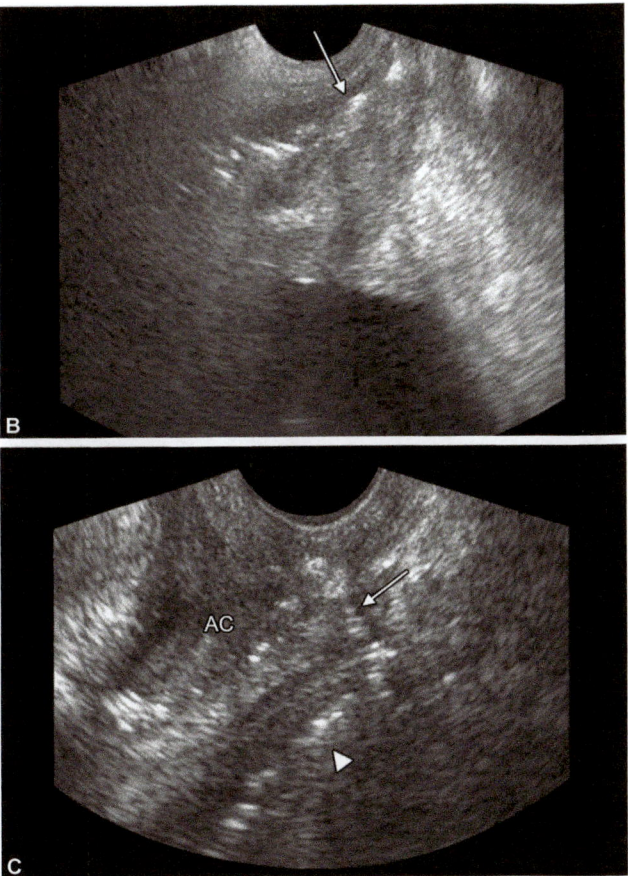

FIGS. 6.31A AND C: (A) Axial scan of the prostate showing gas in the gland with ring down artifacts. (B) Longitudinal scan shows gas outlining the urethra (arrow). (C) Sagittal scan at the level of anal canal (AC) shows a gas-filled fistulous tract (arrow) between the urethra (arrow head) and the anal canal.

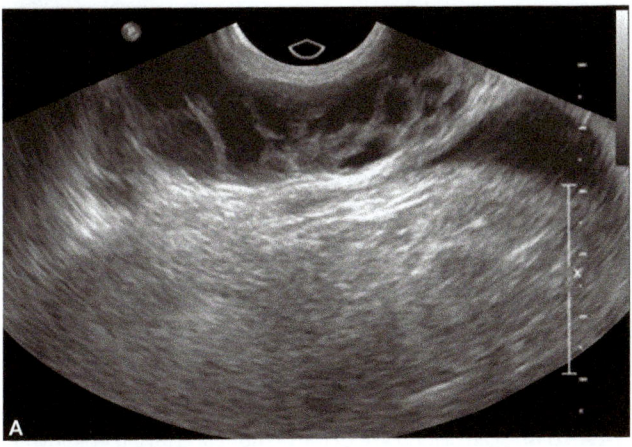

FIGS. 6.32A AND B:

Continued...

Continued...

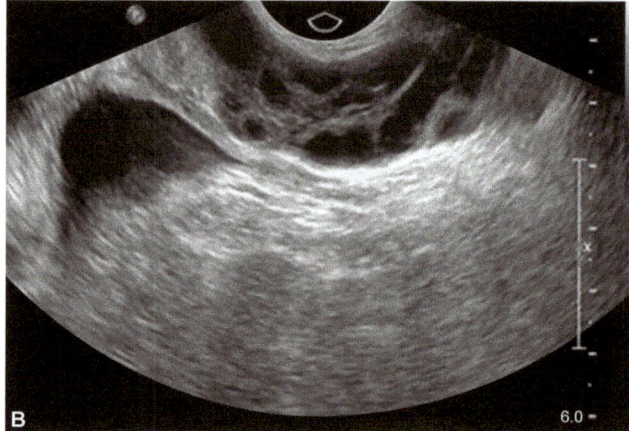

FIGS. 6.32A AND B: Transrectal scans showing the dilated (A) right and (B) left seminal vesicles in a case of obstruction to ejaculatory ducts.

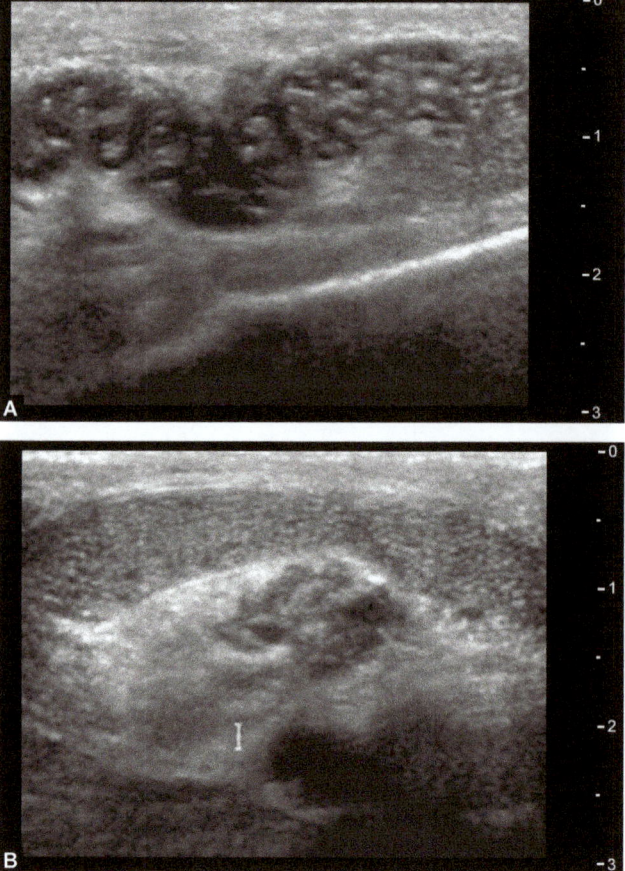

FIGS. 6.33A AND B: Scan of long axis of the (A) right and (B) left epididymis showing dilated tubules of asymmetric nature.

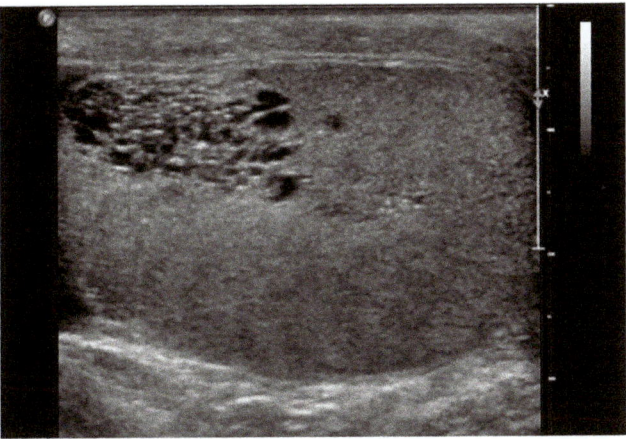

FIG. 6.34: Scan of the testis showing dilated rete testis.

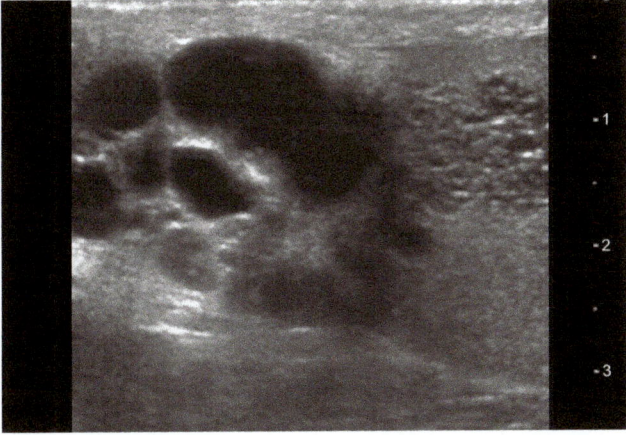

FIG. 6.35: Scan of the testis and epididymis showing multiple epididymal cysts in a case of obstruction to the ejaculatory ducts.

Diffuse enlargement of testis with homogeneous or heterogeneous hypoechoic texture (**Fig. 6.45**) is rarely present.

The differential diagnosis of scrotal tuberculosis are acute nonspecific infection and tumors.

The presence of both epididymal and testicular lesions indicates infection. In case of nonspecific infection, the main clinical feature is that the infection is acute in nature with diffused and homogeneous involvement as compared to the tuberculosis lesion which is of chronic nature with focal heterogeneous.

Quite often, it is difficult to differentiate; however, presence of sinus tract, unresponsiveness to nonspecific antimicrobial agents, and the evidence of tuberculosis in other parts of the genitourinary system can prove to be useful in establishing the difference in both the conditions.

In case of an isolated lesion in the testis, tumor can be ruled out by undertaking biopsy.

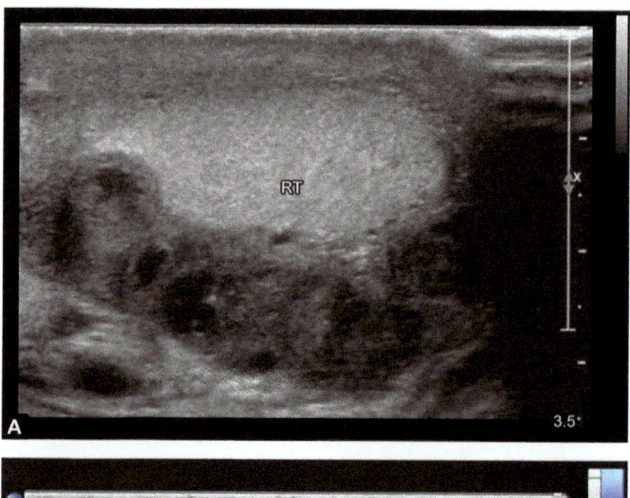
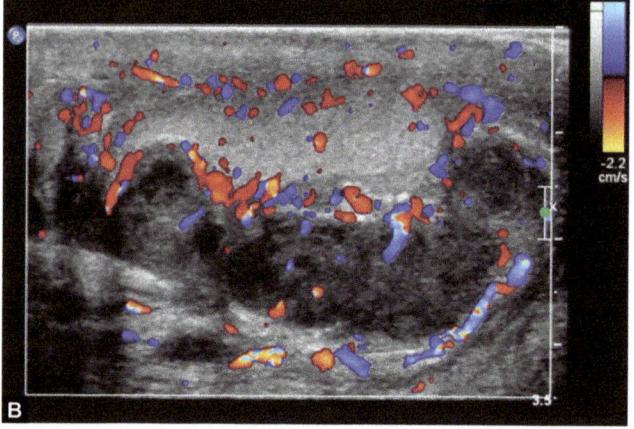

(RT: right testis)

FIGS. 6.36A AND B: (A) Tuberculous epididymitis appearing as a diffusely enlarged heterogeneously hypoechoic epididymis. (B) Color Doppler image showing the flow in the periphery and absence of the flow in the focal lesions.

Tuberculosis of Seminal Vesicles and Vasa Deferentia

Transrectal ultrasonography or TRUS shows small solid seminal vesicles with or without calcifications (**Figs. 6.46A and B**). Presence of single or multiple hypoechoic masses in the vas and the spermatic cord can be visualized (**Fig. 6.47**) along with calcification in vas deferens (**Fig. 6.48**). Major diagnostic feature of tuberculosis are aspermia, fibrosis, and atrophy of the seminal vesicles. In such patients, further evaluation and treatment with assisted reproduction is not required. The main differential diagnosis is congenital absence of vas deferens, which will show an absent seminal vesicle and vas deferens on TRUS and good clinical examination. In rare cases of severe infection, especially in patients with compromised immunity, abscess is present in the small vesicle and usually involve the prostate also (**Figs. 6.49A and B**). Such patients may exhibit symptoms of fever

Sonographic Features of Urinary Tuberculosis

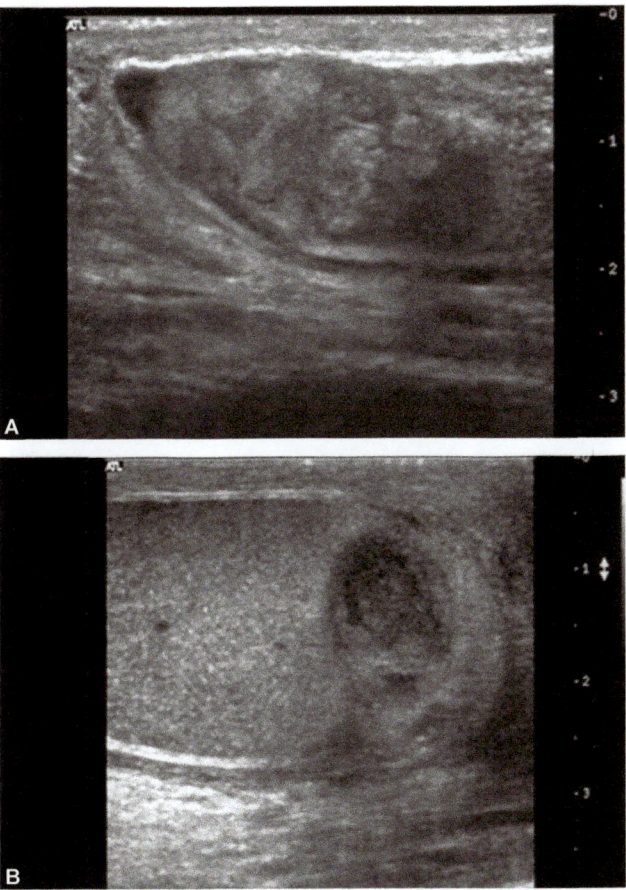

FIGS. 6.37A AND B: Focal nodular heterogeneous lesion of (A) head and (B) tail of epididymis.

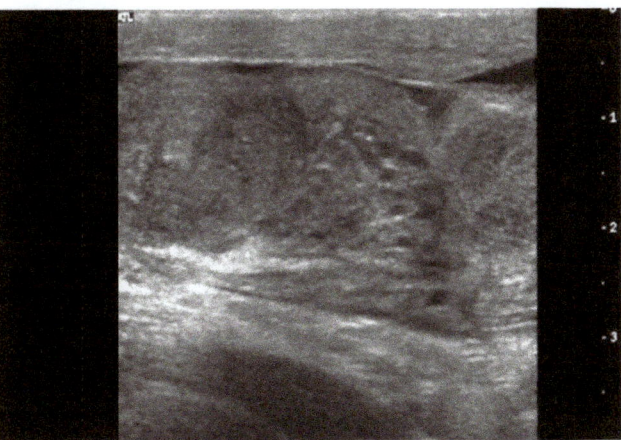

FIG. 6.38: Image shows a diffusely enlarged homogeneously hypoechoic epididymis.

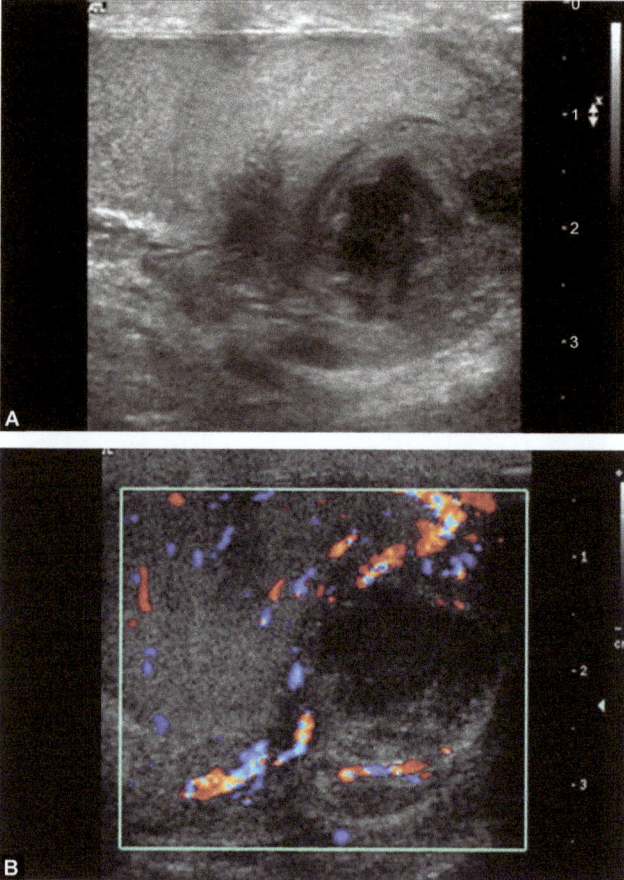

FIGS. 6.39A AND B: (A) Gray scale and (B) color Doppler images of a tuberculous abscess in the tail of epididymis.

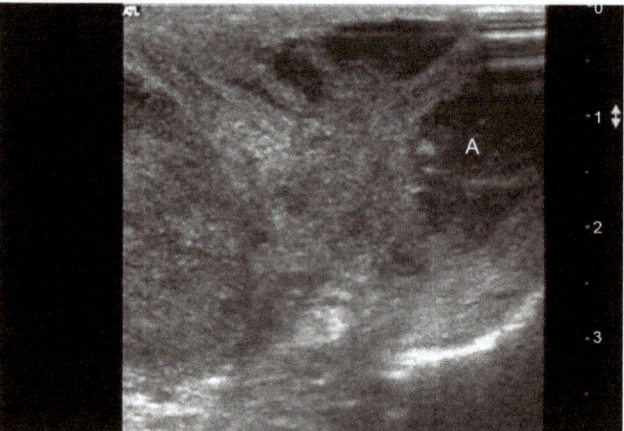

FIG. 6.40: Image showing extension of the tuberculous lesion of the tail of the epididymis into the scrotal wall with an abscess in the wall (A).

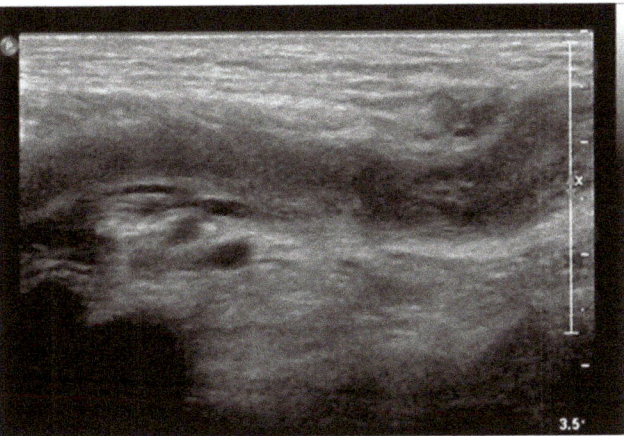

FIG. 6.41: Scan of the scrotum showing an echopoor tract extending from the sinus opening in the wall to the tail of epididymis.

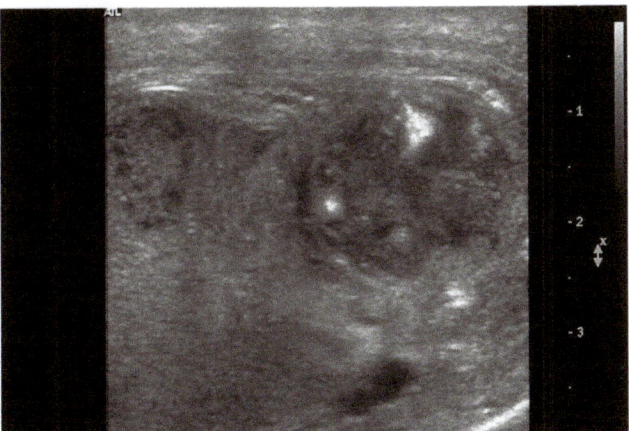

FIG. 6.42: Image showing a focal nodular heterogeneous lesion in the tail of the epididymis with calcifications.

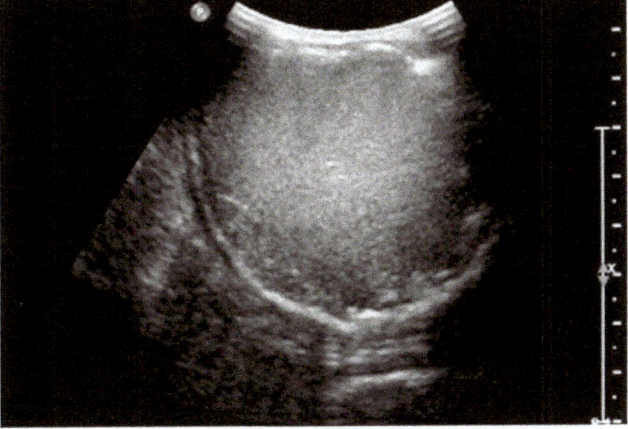

FIG. 6.43: Chronic hydrocele with calcification of the tunica vaginalis.

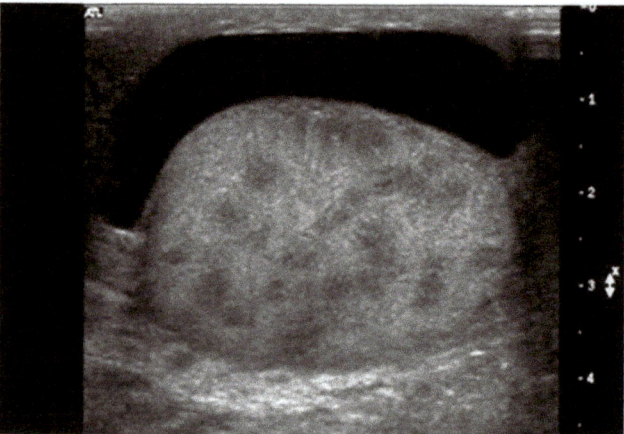

FIG. 6.44: Image showing an enlarged testis with multiple small hypoechoic nodules. There is also hydrocele.

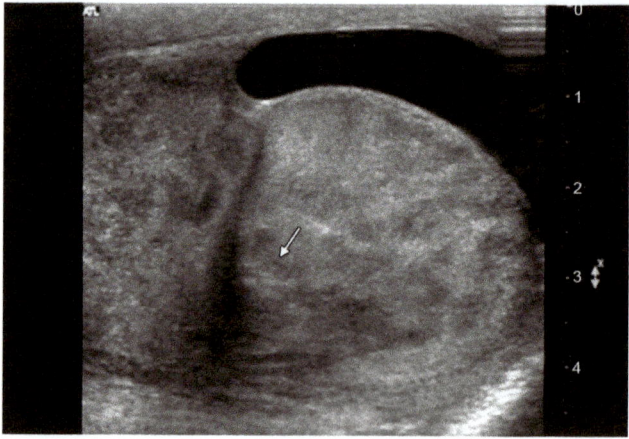

FIG. 6.45: Diffusely enlarged testis with heterogeneous hypoechoic texture with a blurred interface between the testis and the epididymis (arrow).

and irritative voiding symptoms. In these patients, TRUS shows an abscess in the seminal vesicle which can be viewed as an enlarged seminal vesicle filled with fluid and debris in it. Involvement of the prostate and loss of interface between the seminal vesicle and the prostate can also occur along with the thickening of adjacent wall of the urinary bladder. The findings can be imitative of a pyogenic abscess and USG-guided aspiration will be useful in ruling out tuberculosis.

Female Genital Tract Tuberculosis

In female genital tract, the fallopian tube is the primary site of infection; infection mainly spreads by hematogenous route. Most often, it can be caused due to a lymphatic spread

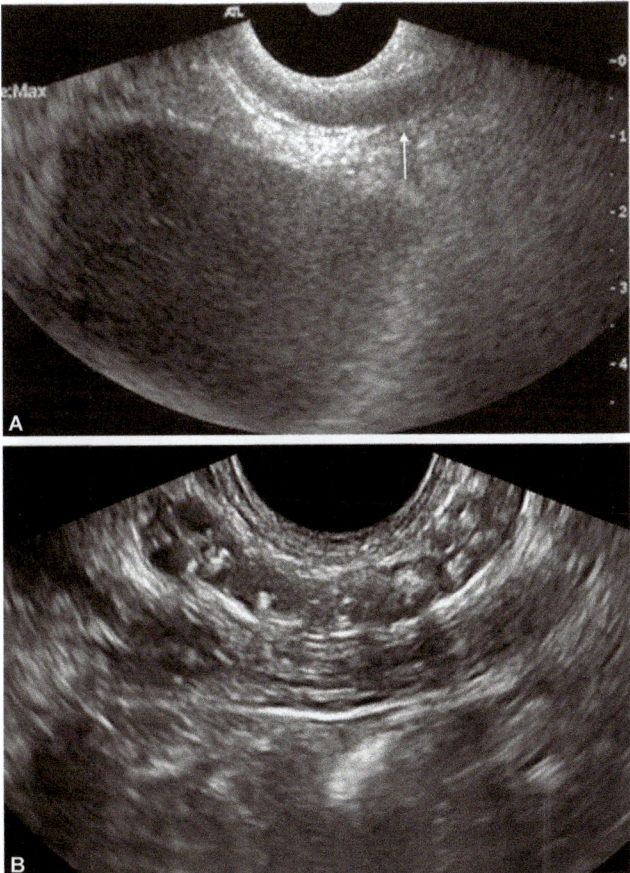

FIGS. 6.46A AND B: (A) Transrectal ultrasound image showing a small, thin, and solid seminal vesicle (arrow). (B) Image showing extensive calcifications in both seminal vesicles.

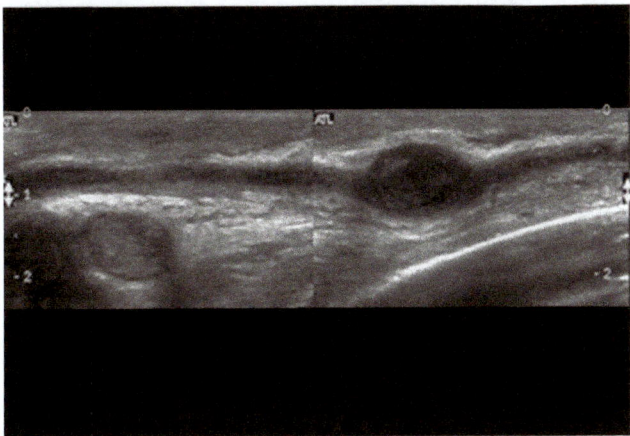

FIG. 6.47: Image showing a hypoechoic mass of the vas deferens in the spermatic cord due to tuberculosis.

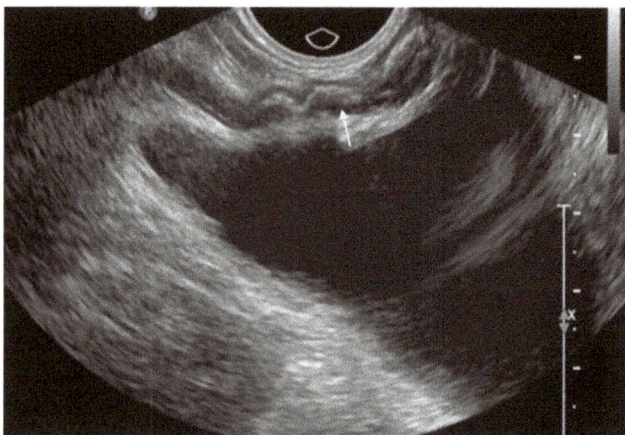

FIG. 6.48: Transrectal ultrasound image showing calcifications in the vas deferens.

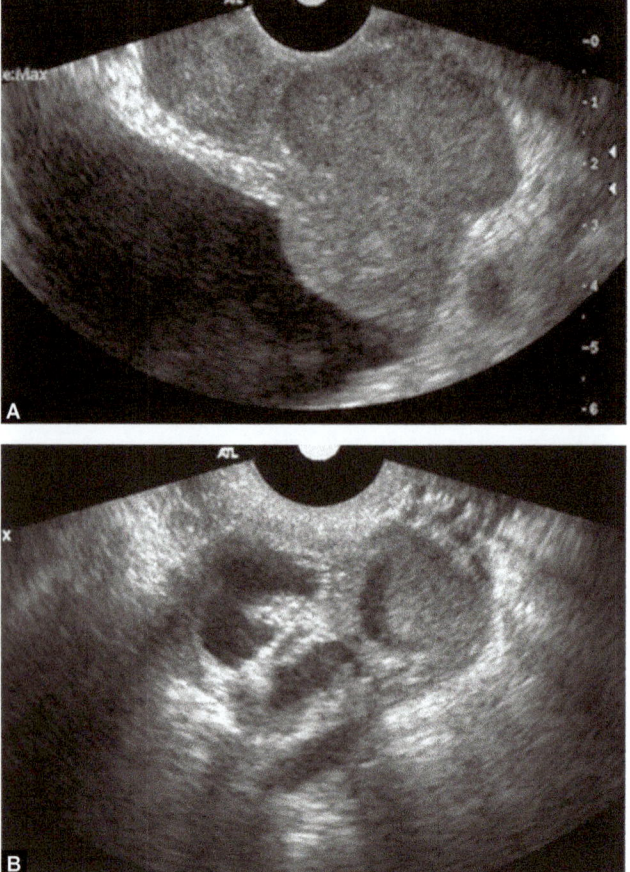

FIGS. 6.49A AND B: Two sections of the seminal vesicle and prostate showing an irregular solid and cystic mass suggestive of an abscess in the seminal vesicle involving the prostate and indenting on the urinary bladder.

from peritoneal implants or as a direct extension from an intestinal lesion. About 94% of women with genital tuberculosis have involvement in the fallopian tubes. There are two types of female pelvic tuberculosis pathologically.
1. *Wet type*: In the "wet" type, ascites is present. Numerous small tubercles cover the viscera and the peritoneum of the parietal wall. In addition to being covered with miliary tubercles on the serosal surface, the fallopian tubes, are often slightly enlarged and distended. As compared to other forms of salpingitis, the fimbriae may be patent. Histology is typical of tuberculosis with tubercle formation, multinucleated giant cells, and epithelioid reaction in the tubal wall and mucosa. Frank caseation is present in advanced cases.
2. *The "Dry" or the adhesive type tuberculosis*: It presents as the healed fibrotic end result of the wet ascitic pattern. The pelvic organs reveal evidence of tuberculous salpingitis with the following:
   - Enlargement of the tubes
   - Occasionally pyosalpingitis
   - Tubo-ovarian abscess formation

On sonography, ascites is often septated with lattice-like appearance (**Fig. 6.50A**). Ascetic fluid may contain echogenic particles; thickening of greater omentum (**Fig. 6.50A**) and parietal as well as visceral peritoneum (**Fig. 6.50B**) may be present. Ascitic fluid may also contain thickened and floating fallopian tubes (**Fig. 6.50C**). With adhesions, the ascites may be loculated with thick septa, imitating a tumor in the ovary or tubo-ovarian abscess (**Fig. 6.51**). In the dry type, the walls of the fallopian tubes are thick (**Figs. 6.52A to C**). It may show distended lumen with irregular thick walls with well-preserved patency on saline infusion sonohysterography. Hydrosalpinx may be present (**Fig. 6.53**). Usually, there is a bilateral involvement of the fallopian tube. Infections as well as cases of ovarian carcinoma also present with most of these features. The occurrence of the combination of these features especially with septated ascites favors tuberculosis. Tuberculosis is confirmed with laparoscopy and biopsy. In case of patient presenting with infertility, sonography can show hydrosalpinx. Saline infusion sonohysterography may either be remarkable for a tubal block or an abnormal fallopian tubes, in case where endovaginal sonography does not reveal any abnormality.

Endometrial Tuberculosis

In 50% of patients with tubal tuberculosis, there is an involvement of uterine endometrium as an extension of disease from the fallopian tube. Nearly 11.5% of the patients with pulmonary tuberculosis exhibit the same. The pathology involves granulomas and caseation necrosis. Adhesions and calcification lead to shrunken cavity in later stages. Infertility (45-55%), menstrual disturbances (20%), or amenorrhea are clinical presentations in patients. Few patients remain asymptomatic. Saline infusion sonohysterography is the technique of sonography, which reveals some features of endometrial tuberculosis. The features which suggest tuberculosis are:
- Irregular contour of endometrium
- Endometrial polyp
- Synechia
- Scarred cavity (**Figs. 6.54A and B**)

Histological diagnosis can be established by dilatation and curettage or hysteroscopic biopsy. Tiny specks of bright echoes in the endometrium are indicative of endometrial calcification (**Fig. 6.55**). If extensive, it can imitate endometrial osseous metaplasia.

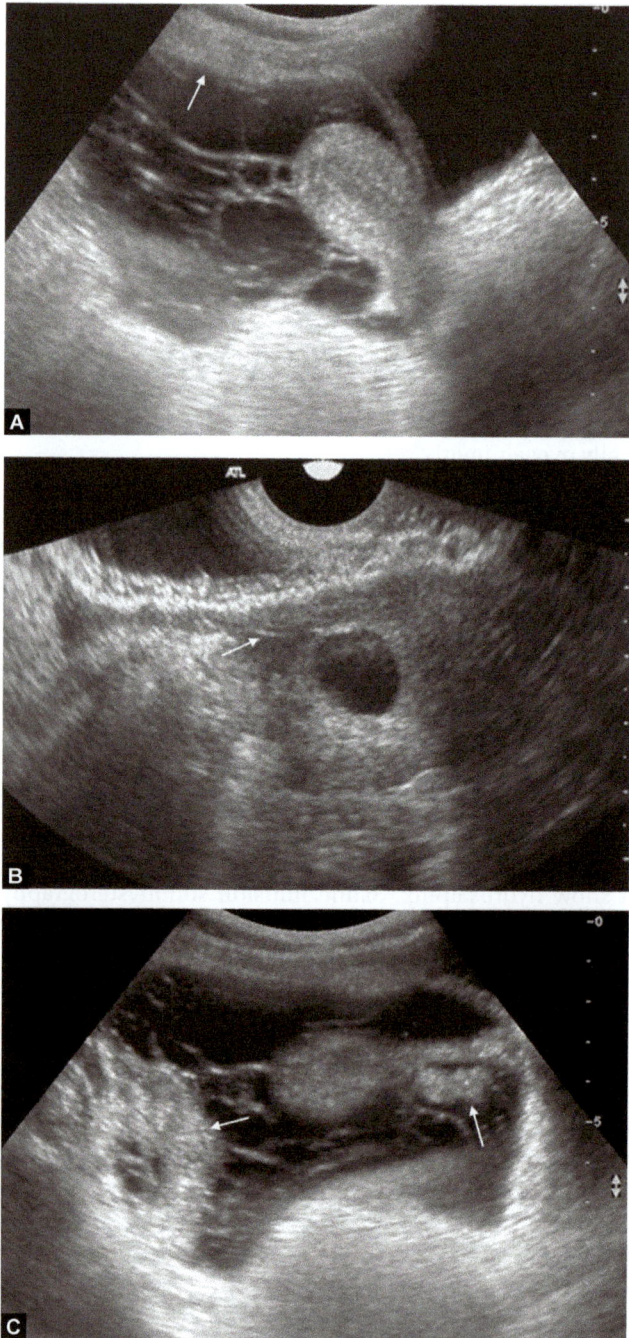

FIGS. 6.50A TO C: (A) Sagittal scan of the pelvis showing septated ascites with a lattice-like appearance with thick greater omentum (arrow). (B) Endovaginal scan showing free fluid in the pelvis with thickening of peritoneum (arrow). (C) Transverse scan shows the irregularly thickened fallopian tubes on both sides (arrows).

Sonographic Features of Urinary Tuberculosis

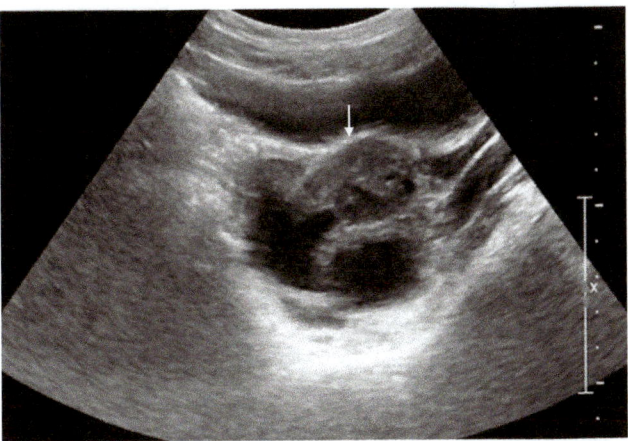

FIG. 6.51: Oblique scan of the adnexa showing a tubo-ovarian abscess (arrow) due to tuberculosis.

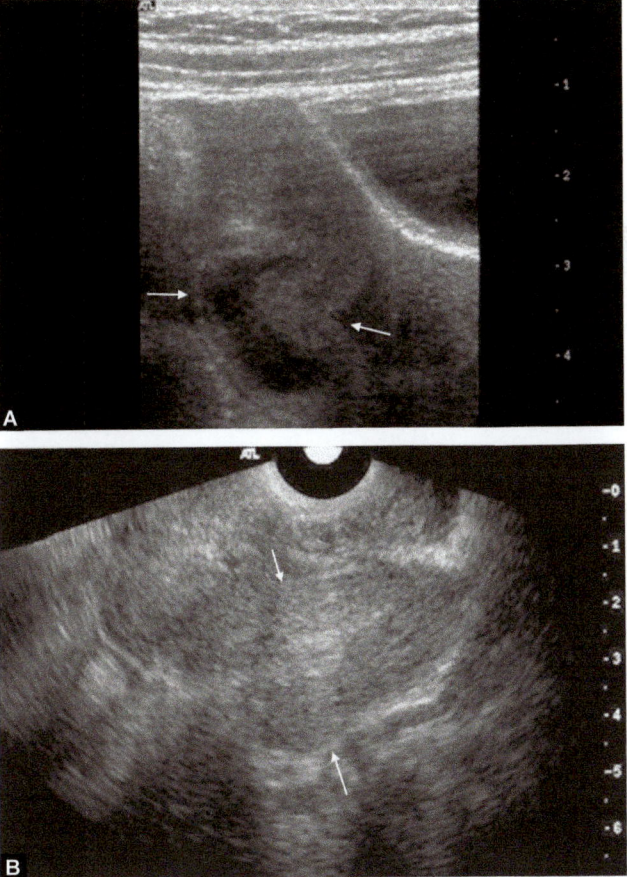

FIGS. 6.52A TO C:

Continued...

Continued...

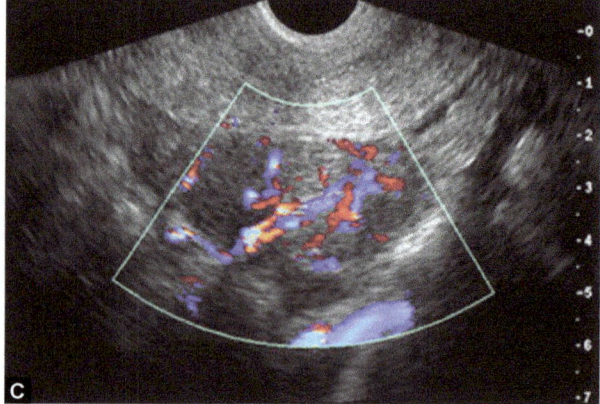

FIGS. 6.52A TO C: Dry type of pelvic tuberculosis. (A) High-resolution sonography abdominal image showing a thick-walled fluid distended fallopian tube (arrows). (B) Endovaginal image showing the markedly thick-walled fallopian tube (arrows). (C) Color Doppler image showing hyperemia of the fallopian tube.

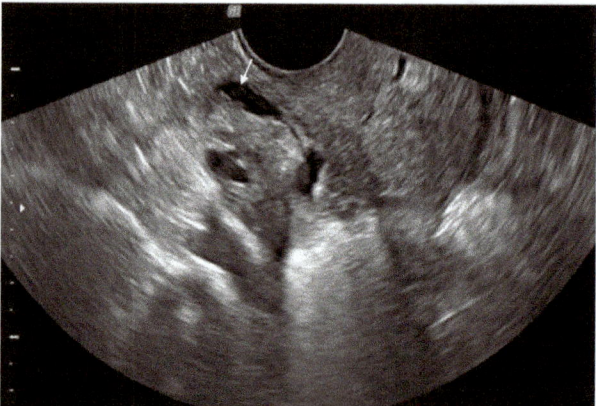

FIG. 6.53: Image shows hydrosalpinx with thick walls (arrows) due to tuberculosis.

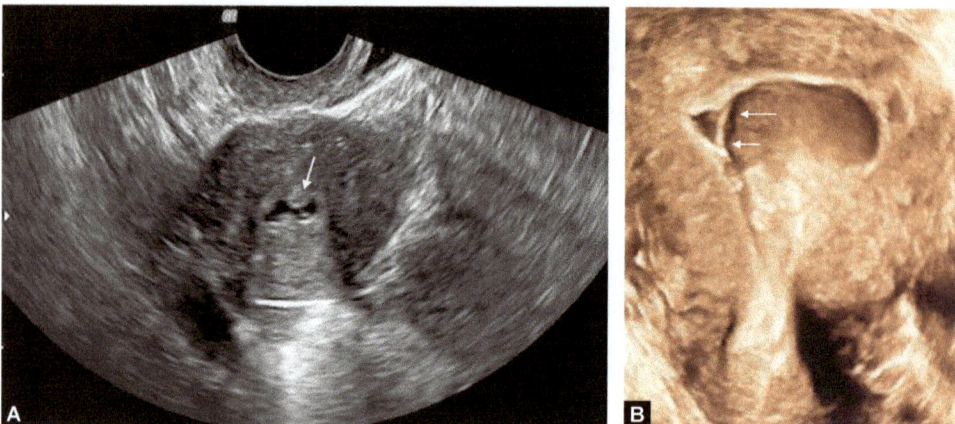

FIGS. 6.54A AND B: (A) Saline infusion sonohysterography image showing irregular contour of the endometrium with a polyp (arrow). (B) Four-dimensional image of saline infusion sonohysterography showing a synechia (arrows).

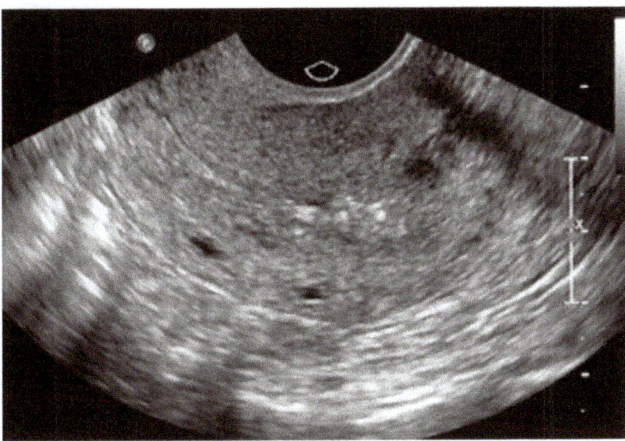

FIG. 6.55: Longitudinal scan of the uterus showing punctuate calcifications in the endometrium.

REFERENCE

1. The section of urinary tuberculosis is adapted from the article by the author: Vijayaraghavan SB, Kandasamy SV, Arul M, Prabhakar M, Dhinakaran CL, Palanisamy R. Spectrum of high-resolution sonographic features of urinary tuberculosis. J Ultrasound Med. 2004;23(5):585-94, with the permission of American Institute of Ultrasound Medicine.

CHAPTER 7

Outline of Medical and Surgical Management

Sujata Patwardhan

TREATMENT: MEDICAL

The reasons for using multiple drugs in treatment of tuberculosis (TB) are as follows:
- The TB bacilli will be in the different microenvironments in the same host having different metabolic needs and replication speeds.
- The drugs used are either bactericidal or bacteriostatic.
- Some drugs act better on replicating bacteria and some on dormant bacteria.
- Each drug has different penetrations in different tissues and *Mycobacterium tuberculosis*, being a slowly replicating bacteria, requires multiple drug therapy.

Treatment is started after routine investigations for complete blood count (CBC), liver function test (LFT), renal function test (RFT), human immunodeficiency virus (HIV), and Hepatitis B and C. If culture is positive, then the information should be utilized to prescribe culture-sensitive drugs. First-line anti-TB treatment starts with isoniazid (INH), rifampicin, ethambutol, and pyrazinamide, which is a standard 6 months' course in given with an intensive phase of 2 months and continuation phase of 4 months. It is necessary to emphasize the following points to patients:
- The nature and duration of treatment
- Importance of adherence to treatment
- The need to complete the treatment
- Consequences of irregular treatment or premature cessation of treatment
- Possible side effect of drugs
- *Mechanism of transmission of disease:* Close family members should be include in counseling about family planning.
- All patients with results of culture, smears, CBNAAT (cartridge-based nucleic acid amplification test) are communicated to DTD (District TB officer) and enrolled in "Nikshay" scheme.
- Patient must be counseled for prevention of transmission, especially if genitourinary (GU) Koch's is associated with pulmonary Koch's.
- History should include close contact with patient of multidrug-resistant (MDR) TB, close contact of patient who died on TB treatment, and close contact of patient who failed TB treatment.

- Vulnerable groups have to be identified which include patients attending HIV OPD's, substance abuse including smoking, patients with diabetes, malignancy, dialysis, immunosuppression, patients in prison, deaddiction center, old age homes, etc.

Although 6 months is a standard duration, there are clinical scenarios where the duration is extended:
- Extensive TB with pockets of infection
- Concurrent smear-positive cavitary pulmonary TB
- Concurrent CNS involvement
- Patient unable to take pyrazinamide for first 2 months

Because of the various clinical scenarios which may arise, special advice from DTD should be taken if you plan to deviate from the standard treatment protocol.

Pyridoxine is given along with AKI to prevent INH-induced peripheral neuropathy. Patients with preexisting liver disease are monitored with frequent LFTs. Patients on ethambutol may have hepatic toxicity and are advised to abstain from alcohol or hepatotoxic drugs. Visual activity and red–green perception should be monitored for patients on ethambutol.

Response to treatment should be evaluated at 8 weeks in terms of improvement in symptoms, resolution of symptoms, and renal function tests.

Patients with radiological evidence obstruction may treat with new fibrosis and worsening of urinary obstruction. Repeat imaging may be indicated in such patients. Culture-positive patients at diagnosis may be subjected to repeat culture at 8 weeks and end of 6 months. Worsening obstruction may have to be diverted. Surgical procedures can be initiated after 6 weeks as the active inflammation is thought to subside.

Role of Steroids

The role of steroids is not very clear and was utilized to avail the anti-inflammatory effects of steroids. They are indicated in TB meningitis, peritonitis, pericarditis, and few forms of pulmonary TB.

The role of steroids to prevent ureteral strictures in genitourinary tuberculosis (GUTB) has not been established in literature.

Patients who present with new lesions of TB after 6 months of standard first-line anti-TB drugs are subjected to specific cultures and sensitivity, and if the cultures are negative for drug resistance, standard 6 months' first-line therapy is repeated.

Second-line agents are given only if the culture are showing resistance to first-line drugs (bacteriologically positive after initial course of AKT), contact with MDR TB (during or before) the treatment of first-line AKT (**Tables 7.1** and **7.2**).

Surgical Management

In our experience, the number of patients who require surgical intervention during their course of treatment for GUTB disease are 100% (at a tertiary care center); however, Wang et al. have reported that 55% of their patients required surgical intervention.

Diversion

Sepsis and uremia would be indications mentioned in literature for prompt relief of obstruction. However, urinary diversion is not be required as emergency procedure but rather required as an elective procedure in our experience. In majority of instances an elective ureteral stenting or PCN can be done to prevent further loss of renal function and

TABLE 7.1: Antituberculous first-line drugs.

Drug	Recommended dose		Adverse effects
	Daily	Intermittent	
Isoniazid (INH)	5 mg/kg	10 mg/kg	Hepatotoxicity, peripheral neuritis, (pyridoxine prevents it), rashes, arthralgia
Rifampin	10 mg/kg	10 mg/kg	Hepatotoxicity, flu-like symptoms, drug interactions (microsomal enzyme inducer), cutaneous syndrome (flushing and pruritus), abdominal syndrome (nausea, vomiting, and cramps), respiratory syndrome (breathlessness may be associated with shock, and collapse)
Pyrazinamide	25 mg/kg	35 mg/kg	Hepatotoxicity, hyperuricemia, arthralgia, flushing, and rashes
Ethambutol	15 mg/kg	30 mg/kg	Loss of visual acuity, color vision, field defects, optic neuritis (should not be used below 6 years of age)
Streptomycin	15 mg/kg	15 mg/kg	Renal damage, vestibular and cochlear toxicity

TABLE 7.2: Antituberculous second-line drugs.

Drug	Recommended dose	Adverse effects
Capreomycin	15 mg/kg IM or IV (maximum 1 g)	Vestibular and cochlear toxicity, Nephrotoxicity, dyselectrolytemia
Kanamycin	15 mg/kg IM or IV (maximum 1 g)	Nephrotoxicity, ototoxicity
Amikacin	15 mg/kg IM or IV (maximum 1 g)	Nephrotoxicity, ototoxicity
Cycloserine	10–15 mg/kg in divided oral doses	Psychiatric symptoms, tremors, sleepiness, headache, convulsions
Ethionamide	15–20 mg/kg in divided oral doses	Abdominal upset, nausea, vomiting, hepatitis, peripheral or optic neuritis, mental disturbances, impotence
Levofloxacin	500–1,000 mg oral or IV	GI disturbances, QT prolongation, tendinitis or tendon rupture
Moxifloxacin	400 mg oral or IV	GI disturbances, QT prolongation, tendinitis or tendon rupture
Aminosalicylic acid	8–12 g in divided oral doses	Anorexia, nausea, epigastric pain, hypothyroidism, hepatotoxicity
Linezolid	600 mg BD oral	Bone marrow suppression, peripheral neuritis, optic neuritis, hepatotoxicity
Bedaquiline	400 mg oral	Headache, arthralgia, QT prolongation, hepatitis
Rifabutin		Uveitis, granulocytopenia, myalgia, GI intolerance
Clarithromycin	500 mg BD oral	Ototoxicity

(GI: gastrointestinal; IM: intramuscular; IV: intravenous)

prior to reconstructive surgery. Both, Double J (DJ) stent or percutaneous nephrostomy (PCN) can be done. Though a DJ stent may be preferred, but at times DJ stenting may not be possible due to complete obstruction. PCN can be done and kept until healing after surgery is documented.

As more than one infundibulum get involved in the fibrosis, PCN may have to be placed in more than one site in same kidney. It has been mentioned in literature that DJ stenting is successful in 41% of cases.[1] Contrast injection during placement of PCN should not be under pressure to avoid dissemination of infection.

Minimally Invasive Management

Strictures in tuberculosis are characterized by tuberculous ulceration and subsequent fibrosis. The fibrosis is usually dense and hence results of endoscopic management is suboptimal.

Strictures, which are formed during medical management, are managed by early stenting and do not required further surgical management.[2]

Balloon dilatation by antegrade or retrograde access has been utilized for management of tuberculosis strictures of the ureter.[3] Patients having evidence of obstruction would require follow-up imaging during medical management. It is necessary to document that there is no increasing obstruction during medical management after 6–8 weeks of starting AKT.

Patients undergoing endoscopic management also require follow-up imaging after the stents are removed, as some strictures worsen during healing process. Failure to improve after 6 weeks of medical management or failure to improve after endoscopic interventions are indications for definitive surgical management. However, the indications for endoscopic interventions are few.

Surgical Management

Nephrectomy

Indications for nephrectomy are nonfunctioning kidney, putty or calcified kidney, persistent fistula associated with nonfunctioning or calcified kidney, medically resistant hypertension with nonfunctioning kidney, and recurrent tuberculosis despite optimum medical management.

Traditionally, open surgical approach has been utilized for nephrectomy in tuberculosis, this is because of the extensive fibrosis, granulation, and caseous cavities which may be encountered in the perinephric fat, perinephric space, and surface of the kidney. Case is taken to avoid entry into the pleura and peritoneum and avoid dissemination. Renal artery and vein are preferably ligated separately. Ureters are usually taken as much as possible through the incision, but it is not necessary to remove the ureter up to the ureterovesical (VU) junction.

Through various authors have advocated laparoscopic nephrectomy and reported good outcomes, the procedure of choice would depend upon expertise of operating surgeon. If the nephrectomy is associated with drainage of perinephric or psoas abscess, retroperitoneal open approach is ideal.

When the nephrectomy is done for fistula/sinus, it may be kept in mind that the perinephric space may be involved with multiple sinuses and adhesions and open surgical approach is better.

Surgery for Infundibulum

Since TB can involve more than one infundibulum of the kidney, intrarenal surgery is almost impossible when multiple infundibuli are involved. A very small and narrow pelvis in tuberculosis is another reason why reconstructive procedures of renal pelvis are difficult. A ureterocalicostomy may be done, provided the dependent calyx is freely communicating with upper calyces.

Pelvic and Ureteric Strictures

The pelvis in tuberculosis is usually narrow, less capacious and hiked up and may not be adequate for a good Anderson-Hyne's pyeloplasty for upper ureteric strictures. The length and degree of stricture, vascular supply of the ureter, and the presence of calcification in the ureters are factors which would decide the surgical procedure.

Impaired renal function in this setting of long dense upper ureteric stricture may lead to a nephrectomy, lower ureteric strictures are more common and can be managed by ureteroneocystostomy.

Ureterocalicostomy is an option when the lower calyx is not diseased and is freely communicating with entire pelvicalyceal (PC) system. Davis intubated ureterostomy may be done for midureteric strictures and short segment upper ureteric stricture after adhesiolysis and using available omentum to prevent further adhesions and fibrosis.

Boari flap may be utilized to bridge gap of 10–15 cm along with psoas hitch. However, bladder capacity needs to be measured before as contracted bladder may not allow flap creation. Ileal interposition can be done for multiple strictures of ureter; however, intraoperative bowel needs to be evaluated for gastrointestinal tuberculosis.

Bladder Surgery

For severe frequency, nocturia, urgency, pain, hematuria, and capacity <100 mL, bladder augmentation is an option. It may be performed utilizing ileum, ileocecum, or sigmoid colon.

Suturing the ileum to thick-walled bladder may be difficult at times and a thimble bladder <20 mL can be managed by orthotopic bladder substitution.[4]

The patient should be explained the complication of surgery and need for CSIC. Bladder neck contracture is best managed by bladder neck incision. Tuberculous fistulae with the urethra should be first managed by prolonged first-line chemotherapy and suprapubic diversion. Rectourethral fistulae are also managed in the similar way and the resulting strictures after 9–12 months of AKT are managed by end-to-end anastomosis by progressive perineal approach with excision of fistula.

Vesicovaginal fistulas (VVFs) are seen in tuberculosis. The fistulae may be multiple, large, and may require bladder augmentation before VVF closure. Simultaneous use of ileum for augmentation of the bladder and for vaginal reconstruction has been reported.[5]

Cystectomy with Ileal Conduit

In our experience, five patients with creatinine >3 mg/dL with thimble bladder and lower ureteric stricture underwent cystectomy with ileal conduit for preservation of residual renal function and diversion. It is important to note that conduit was a short segment approximately 5 cm in length, just adequate to both ureters to be implanted and just adequate stoma to be created. Patients were advised overnight drainage with Foley catheter, all with intention to prevent metabolic complications.

Rat Tail Anastomosis

A segment of 5-6 cm of ileum can be utilized for reimplantation of both the ureters and the lower end anastomosis to dome of detrusor. This procedure is useful when there are bilateral long ureteric strictures and bladder capacity is either adequate or small.

Permanent Diversion

In our experience of five patients who had multiple ureteric stricture and unwilling for surgery, patients continued to follow up with multiple unilateral or bilateral nephrostomies and did not option for surgical management.

Genital Surgery

Epididymectomy can be done with sparing of the testis and testicular blood supply for tuberculosis involving the epididymis and not resolving with medical management. If the testes are infected completely, an orchidectomy can be done special consent regarding fertility issues should be documented before surgery.

REFERENCES

1. Ramanathan R, Kumar A, Kapoor R, Bhandari M. Relief of urinary tract obstruction in tuberculosis to improve renal function. Analysis of predictive factors. Br J Urol. 1998;81(2):199-205.
2. Shin KY, Park HJ, Lee JJ, Park HY, Woo YN, Lee TY. Role of early endourologic management of tuberculous ureteral strictures. J Endourol. 2002;16(10):755-8.
3. Murphy DM, Fallon B, Lane V, O'Flynn JD. Tuberculous stricture of ureter. Urology. 1982;20(4):382-4.
4. Hemal AK, Aron M. Orthotopic neobladder in management of tubercular thimble bladders: initial experience and long-term results. Urology. 1999;53(2):298-301.
5. Sujata K. Patwardhan et al. Simultaneous bladder and vaginal reconstruction using ileum in complicated vesicovaginal fistula. Indian J Urol. 2008;24(3):348-51.

CHAPTER 8

Surgery Outcomes

Nitin Kekre, Anuj Deep Dangi

HISTORICAL INSIGHTS INTO THE ROLE OF SURGERY FOR URINARY TUBERCULOSIS

Tuberculosis (TB) is a systemic infection which usually manifests with the combination of predominantly local and less often systemic symptoms (e.g., fever, weight loss, and anorexia). Local symptoms arise due to the reactivation of the dormant focus of TB. The outcome of the infection depends on interaction between host immunity, bacterial virulence, and bacterial load at a given time. Medical therapeutics (including chemotherapy and surgery) has the potential to alter outcomes by changing the delicate balance of interaction between host immunity and the pathogen.

Specifically in the context of urinary TB, in an era before the advent of effective chemotherapeutics, nephrectomy was done in an attempt to treat urinary TB. Its efficacy remained controversial as it had not been proven beyond doubt that it was successful in altering the natural course of events.[1] During the initial years of introduction of chemotherapy, extirpative surgery (especially nephrectomy) was used as an adjunct to improve therapeutic efficacy.[2] As multidrug chemotherapy became the norm, its potency increased as well with the following far-reaching consequences:

- The once fatal disease became treatable and the focus shifted from saving life to managing other long-term consequences of the disease, i.e., to save the function of the involved organ.[3]
- The question concerning the need for nephrectomy in addition to multidrug therapy became less relevant as clinical scenarios involving unresolved pathological processes after effective multidrug therapy became relatively rare.
- The realization that obstruction of urinary conduits in the kidney were responsible for the destruction of "twice as many renal lobes" as compared to direct tubercular involvement, paved the way for reconstructive surgical procedures dealing with such obstruction.[4] Probably, the chemotherapeutic agents enhanced healing with fibrosis which caused more obstruction-related renal unit damage. Hence, reconstructive surgeries established themselves as an important tool in the treatment armamentarium for urinary TB.

The main aims and objectives of reconstructive surgery were:
- Preservation of renal function by providing adequate drainage and storage of urine at a safe pressure.
- To improve the quality of life in cases of intractable lower urinary tract symptoms arising due to tubercular involvement of the lower urinary tract (bladder, prostate, or urethra).
- To drain nonresolving symptomatic abscess/collections in spite of multidrug therapy.

Preservation of renal function should be the overriding principle amongst the above-stated goals. Decreasing renal function has been shown to be associated with increased mortality,[5] which implies that it is an important parameter which determines long-term survival. Managing quality of life issues, therefore, assumes second importance. Clinical indications for speleotomy or partial nephrectomy with pyelolysis have become rare. Having understood this background, it seems rational to use renal function of the concerned renal unit as the primary yardstick for measuring the success or failure of these reconstructive procedures.

At this point, we would like to bring to the attention of the reader the natural history of urinary TB as documented by Harris et al. They reported that "patients with small renal lesions do not invariably progress to complete destruction of the kidney but may survive." Thus, in some patients, the natural course of events entails slow progression of renal destruction sometimes over decades, even in the absence of surgical or medical treatment.[1] This makes the evaluation of outcomes of reconstruction even more difficult, as they should ideally be compared to the outcome of renal units that were not subjected to medical or surgical treatment. No such comparative data exists and is unlikely to be available in the near future due to obvious ethical reasons, so most of the outcomes reported below would be without comparison to the natural history of disease, but this fact should be borne in mind while interpreting the existing literature.

TIMING AND PREREQUISITES OF RECONSTRUCTIVE SURGICAL PROCEDURES

The final outcome of reconstructive surgery depends on multimodality therapy in addition to host and pathogen factors. It would be ideal to standardize all other factors to the extent practically possible, in order to assess the outcomes of reconstructive surgery alone. In this context, it would be important to discuss the timing and prerequisites of reconstructive surgery. As has been alluded to in the introductory section, once diagnosis of urinary TB is made, multidrug antitubercular therapy is the mainstay of treatment. Baseline renal function and drainage is assessed with the help of various imaging modalities (IVP, CT urography, or radionucleotide scintigraphy) along with serum creatinine-based global renal function assessment. If clinically indicated, initial urinary diversion procedures in the form of percutaneous nephrostomy or double J stent are done. The reassessment of renal unit function and drainage are carried out after 3-4 weeks of intensive phase of multidrug antitubercular therapy. At this point, the decision is made to offer the reconstructive procedure if the involved renal unit is functioning and obstruction is amenable to surgical reconstruction. This procedure is usually undertaken 6-8 weeks into the intensive phase of antitubercular therapy. This protocol was initially adopted and popularized by Gow et al., and very little has been changed over the last four decades as far as this protocol is concerned.[6]

This protocol assumes that the patient is clinically responding to the antitubercular therapy administered. In the present era, especially in cases infected with multidrug-resistant mycobacteria, patients may not respond to the empirical antitubercular therapy instituted while awaiting final culture and sensitivity reporting. In such a scenario, reconstructive procedures should be withheld until drug sensitivity reporting is instituted and appropriate clinical response is achieved. Meanwhile, if indicated, drainage can be done by double J stent or percutaneous nephrostomy tubes. The World Health Organization recommends repeating urine acid-fast bacilli smears at the end of 2 months of intensive phase chemotherapy in case they were positive at diagnosis. This would document the microbiological response to treatment.

Since we would be dealing with reconstructive procedures, a detailed discussion on the need for nephrectomy would be beyond the scope of this discussion; however, interested readers would do well to consult the following references for differing views on the need for nephrectomy for nonfunctioning kidneys along with effective antitubercular therapy.[7-10]

INDICATIONS FOR RECONSTRUCTIVE SURGICAL PROCEDURES

One way to list the surgical procedures is to enumerate them by the anatomical organ they deal with.

Procedures Described for the Kidney and Ureter

- *Speleotomy, cavernotomy, partial nephrectomy, or heminephrectomy:* For removal of progressively enlarging renal calcification associated with renal dysfunction, drainage of nonresolving symptomatic renal collections/abscesses (**Fig. 8.1**) or in some cases to release a kinked renal pelvis so as to improve drainage of the remaining kidney (**Fig. 8.2**).[3] Though these procedures are not exactly reconstructive surgeries, they aimed to preserve renal function and improve drainage and hence will be discussed here.

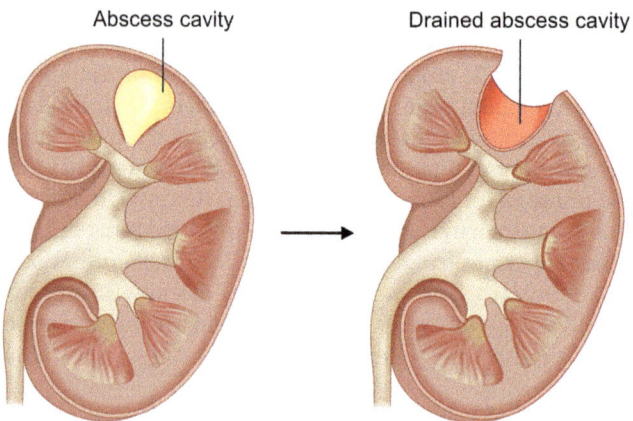

FIG. 8.1: Line diagram showing the speleotomy procedure.

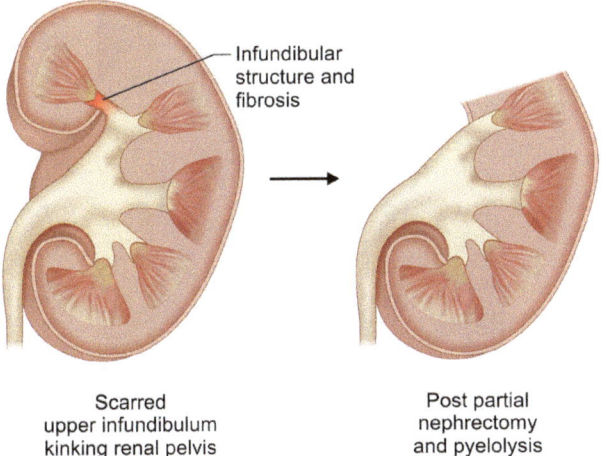

FIG. 8.2: Line diagram showing partial nephrectomy with pyelolysis.

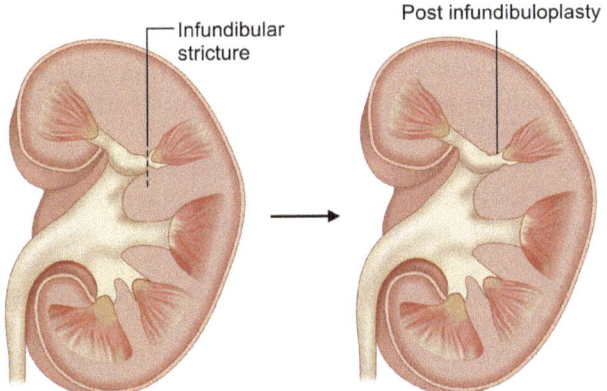

Infundibular repair done by Heineke-Mikukuez principle

FIG. 8.3: Line diagram showing infundibuloplasty.

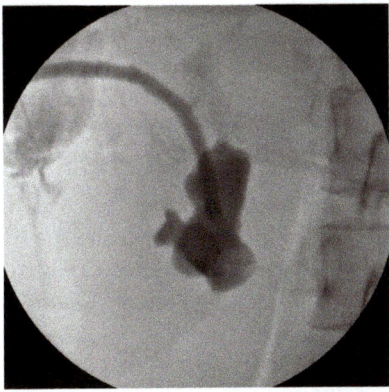

FIG. 8.4: Nephrostogram showing the pelvicalyceal anatomy of kidney prior to reconstruction with ileocalicostomy.

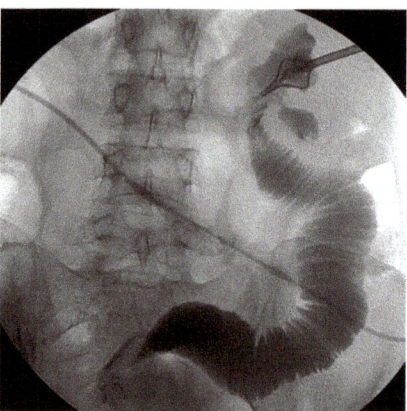

FIG. 8.5: Same renal unit as shown in Figure 8.4, post ileocalicostomy nephrostogram.

- *Renal infundibuloplasty/calicorrhaphy:* When infundibular stenosis (**Fig. 8.3**) is the primary site of obstruction, it is commonly associated with renal pelvic and/or ureteric involvement, and may require procedures such as ureterocalicostomy or ileal ureter with infundibuloplasty (**Figs. 8.4 and 8.5**).
- *Pyeloureteric anastomosis:* For isolated pelviureteric junction stricture.
- *Ureterocalicostomy:* Indicated in cases of failed pyeloureterostomy or offered initially if the renal pelvis is also cicatrized and unusable along with pelviureteric junction stricture.
- *Ureteroneocystostomy:* In cases of isolated lower ureteric strictures where the bladder is relatively uninvolved and bladder capacity is good.
- *Ileal replacement of ureter* (with upper anastomosis to the renal pelvis or dependent renal calyces): In cases of pan-ureteric or multiple long segment ureteric strictures, usually there may be a concomitantly small renal pelvis which may require anastomosis of the ileal segment to the dilated lower calyces or in rare cases of multiple infundibular strictures, opening the kidney laterally as in the anatrophic pyelolithotomy and anastomosing the ileal segment to the calyces (ileal replacement and lateral infundibuloplasty).[9]
- *Buccal mucosal grafting augmentation of ureteric stricture:* In isolated long upper or midureteric stricture not amiable to ureteroureterostomy or ileal replacement, buccal mucosal augmentation with omental wrapping has been reported.[11]

Procedures Described for the Bladder and Prostate

- *Bladder augmentation with a bowel segment:* In cases of small, poorly compliant bladder where there is no contraindication to using the bowel segment, e.g., Crohn's disease or ulcerative colitis with good renal reserve (global renal function).
- *Bladder and prostatic substitution with orthotopic bladder:* When bladder capacity is <20 mL.[12]
- *Noncontinent diversions such as ileal conduits:* In cases of small bladder with compromised renal function and inability or unwillingness to perform clean intermittent catheterization.

The prerequisites of bowel interposition for reconstructive procedures is the presence of good renal reserve. For continent diversion, an eGFR (estimated glomerular filtration rate) (using a creatinine-based GFR equation) of >45 mL/min is preferable.[13]

Procedures for the Urethra

Urethroplasty: Depending on the site and length of the urethral stricture

As a prelude to reconstructive surgery, most renal units with upper urinary tract strictures are diverted by double J stents or percutaneous nephrostomies. These diversions serve two important functions: They preserve renal unit function till reconstructive surgery can be offered (allowing medical therapy to sterilize the tissues) and they are effective to some extent in preventing the development of fibrotic obstructing lesions in the urinary tract. Historically, these forms of diversions (double J stenting and percutaneous nephrostomies) were preceded by periodic ureteric dilatation. Historical accounts of the efficacy of ureteric dilatation are well documented and are discussed in the following text.

Ureteric Dilatation

Kerr et al. reported that out of 30 patients with ureteric strictures, 27 did well with single or multiple treatment sessions of ureteric dilatation over a follow-up period varying from 6 months to 12 years. They used pyelography and calibration with endoscopic dilators to decide on success. One patient was reimplanted at 5 years of follow-up and had received 12 dilatations prior to the surgical intervention. The final outcome based on intravenous pyelography (IVP) has been reported as fair. Two patients underwent nephrectomy at 6 months and 5 years of follow-up, respectively for poor function on IVP. Details on the location, length, and caliber of the strictures are not mentioned.[3] Data published a year later showed that out of 34 patients, five had undergone nephrectomy and one ureteric reimplant on follow-up. Thus, 82.3% (28/34) strictures were stabilized after initial dilatations at 6 months to 12 years of follow-up. In the follow-up study, the authors did clarify that strictures subjected to dilatation were lower ureteric strictures. They also added that initial difficult dilatation or poor response to the first dilatation predicted poor outcomes and such patients should be subjected to ureteric reimplant.[14] Patients in whom dilatation is successful are probably those in whom the obstruction is due to mucosal inflammatory edema which resolves after starting ATT or in some rare cases of probable scar remodeling.

OUTCOME OF RECONSTRUCTIVE SURGERIES

Short and Long-term Outcomes

Speleotomy

Kerr et al. reported the outcome of eight cases, which were followed up for 1–8 years: One patient had a temporary fistula for 6 months, which closed subsequently. They did not specifically mention the renal function of the involved renal unit at follow-up, but documented that patients were well at last follow-up and outcomes were excellent, probably pointing to the fact that patients were asymptomatic from the treated renal pathology.[3] A year later, the same group updated their outcomes; out of 12 patients, one patient had a urinoma and fistula in addition to the previously reported fistula. In another patient, they reported renal failure requiring dialysis after deroofing a giant hydrocalyx in a poorly functioning kidney. In this publication, they put forth their definition of success. It included—no recurrence of abscess cavity, correction of distortion of the pelvicalyceal system with good drainage as assessed on intravenous urography (IVU), and arrest in progressive damage of the remaining parenchyma. Based on these criteria, they reported that 83.3% (10/12) patients had functioning parenchyma at a follow-up ranging from 2 to 9 years.[14] Current literature does not report this procedure as the need for it has reduced after the advent of effective chemotherapy such as pyrazinamide which acts intracellularly.[9]

Heminephrectomy/Partial Nephrectomy and Pyelolysis

Twenty patients were followed up for 6 months to 15 years by Kerr et al. after heminephrectomy. Two patients were subjected to nephrectomy as heminephrectomy proved technically impossible. In the remaining 18, IVU findings at follow-up have been mentioned as good for 16 patients, one patient had poor drainage and another had poor concentration of iodinated contrast but good drainage. Four patients complained of loin pain and three patients had lower urinary tract symptoms at follow-up. Preoperative renal function status and the comparison of preoperative and postoperative IVU have not been commented on.[3] A year later, the authors updated their results and found that 77.2% (17/22) had good outcomes at 6 months to 15 years of follow-up. Successful outcome has been defined as preservation of renal function and freedom from infection. Two patients in this group were subjected to late nephrectomy: One at 6 months for persistent hematuria and flank pain and the second at 5 years' follow-up for persistent pain.[14] Kumar et al. reported one patient who was subjected to partial nephrectomy in their series and the kidney became nonfunctional on follow-up. Nonfunction was defined as split renal eGFR <15 mL/min/1.73 m^2.[11] The eGFR was calculated in two steps: (1) global eGFR was calculated using the CKD-EPI (Chronic Kidney Disease Epidemiology Collaboration) creatinine equation (2009) and (2) split function assessment [based on ethylene dicysteine/diethylenetriamine pentaacetate (DTPA) renal nuclear scintigraphy] was used to calculate the proportional eGFR of each renal unit.[5] In this publication, authors put forth the reasons as to why a single renal unit eGFR of 15 mL/min corresponds to irreversible kidney damage that is destined to progress based on existing chronic kidney disease data.[11] Similar to speleotomy, the partial nephrectomy has become a rare procedure and is reported less often in recent series.

Infundibuloplasty

Mochalova et al. have published their experience with four cases of infundibuloplasty. At 15–19 years of follow-up, they considered all four cases as successes. Their definition of success is composite and includes mortality, need for surgical reintervention, restoration of workability, and fertility for females.[15] This procedure is reported rarely and technically difficult to perform. The renal units needing such procedures usually have poorer initial function, which may impact final outcomes.

Ureteropyelostomy

Mochalova et al. have recorded failure in 21.4% (3/14) of renal units undergoing ureteropyelostomy over a follow-up period varying from 8 to 25 years, using a composite definition of success as discussed above.[15]

Kumar et al. reported two cases of "ureteropyelostomy with ureteric reimplant" and found 50% of renal units had eGFR of <15 mL/min at the last follow-up[11] though in this group, both upper and lower ureteric procedures were performed in the same renal units simultaneously (**Figs. 8.6 and 8.7**). Traditionally, performing them simultaneously is considered to render the blood supply of the remaining ureter tenuous. It is important

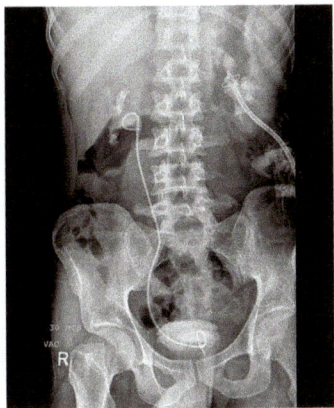

FIG. 8.6: Intravenous pyelography (IVP) showing left renal unit with no drainage beyond pelviureteric junction and has percutaneous nephrostomy in situ, right renal unit has double J stent.

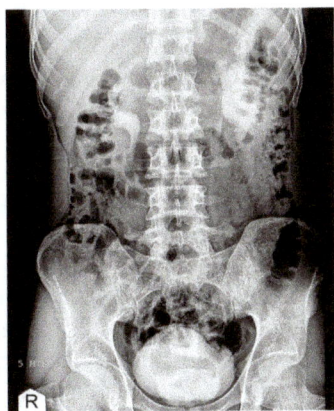

FIG. 8.7: Same left renal unit as shown in Figure 8.6, status simultaneous ureteropyelostomy and ureteric reimplant, 6 months postoperatively.

to note that ureteropyelostomy is more likely to fail than ureteric reimplant of the lower ureter. This data shows that in carefully selected patients, this combination of surgeries is feasible, especially if the function of the renal unit does not support bowel interposition in the form of ileal replacement of the ureter. Where the choice is between nephrectomy and renal preservation with 50% chance of success, this is an acceptable surgical option.

Ureterocalicostomy

Mochalova et al. recorded failure in 18.2% (2/11) renal units undergoing ureterocalicostomies at follow-up ranging from 6 to 18 years, based on a composite definition of success as discussed previously.[15] Kumar et al. reported that 50% (2/4) renal units had an eGFR <15 mL/min at a mean follow-up of 29 months.[11] Ureterocalicostomy is offered in patients where ureteropyelostomy is not feasible or has failed with a small cicatrized renal pelvis.

The outcome of ureterocalicostomy in patients with poor nadir renal function after antitubercular therapy and diversion has been reported by Wagaskar et al.[16] In four patients, whose nadir creatinine ranged between 2 and 3 mg/dL (a creatinine value of 2.5 mg/dL in a 35-year-old gentleman, which was near the mean age reported in the study, would correspond to an eGFR of 30 mL/min/1.73 m^2, based on the CKD-EPI 2009 equation), all four ureterocalicostomies failed. Follow-up duration has not been mentioned in the manuscript; however, it seems that these failures occurred quite early in the follow-up period. They attributed these failures to restructuring of the anastomosis and the presence of multi-infundibular strictures in the involved kidney. Three of these patients had a solitary functioning kidney and were converted to percutaneous nephrostomy as drainage modality, their average nadir creatinine was reported as 2.7 mg%. The fourth patient with two kidneys underwent nephrectomy.[16] Here, the added confounding factor affecting outcome is chronic renal failure, which can result in poor host response. Poor host response can in turn result in a higher degree of parenchymal involvement, poor tissue quality, and possibly ongoing inflammatory process even after the surgery. This information again drives home the point that the place for surgical reconstruction in the sequence of treatment is when the host is in the anabolic phase of recovery from the initial infection.

Ureteric Reimplant/Ureteroneocystostomy

Kerr et al. reported the outcome of 12 patients who underwent ureteric reimplant with follow-up varying from 6 months to 9 years. They report good outcomes based on IVU in all, except one patient who at presentation had uremia and had improved outcome based on IVU assessment postoperatively. Two patients reported infection and loin pain, respectively, at follow-up. They also mentioned their experience with open ureterotomy and T-tube insertion in two patients. In both, outcomes were poor. This was the reason behind them not recommending the procedure.[3] In a later update, these authors reported good outcomes in 13 patients at follow-up ranging from 2 to 15 years. Out of 13 patients, two had a Boari flap used for bridging the gap and eight had a nontunneled anastomosis.[14]

Mochalova et al. reported their experience of 294 surgical procedures of ureteric reimplants using Boari flaps in patients with tubercular lower ureteric strictures; however, the specific details regarding outcomes of this procedure have not been mentioned in the manuscript.[15]

Getahun et al. published their experience with three patients, in all of whom renal functional outcomes were good at a median follow-up of 18 months (range 6–48 months). Good renal function was defined as >25 mL/min/1.73 m^2 based on DTPA clearance on radionucleotide scintigraphy.[17] Kumar et al., who defined poor function of the involved renal unit as eGFR ≤15 mL/min, reported that in patients undergoing unilateral ureteric reimplant, 20% (2/10) renal units had poor function at a mean follow-up of 50.9 months. Four renal units in the bilateral reimplant group had good renal function at a mean follow-up of 43.5 months. Hence, as the follow-up duration becomes longer, a few renal units do lose their function following ureteric reimplant.[11]

Transureteroureterostomies

Mocholova et al. have reported successful outcomes for two transureteroureterostomies performed by them with a follow-up of 6 and 10 years, respectively.[15] This procedure has not been reported by other series. The indication for such a procedure is rare: Isolated unilateral upper ureteric stricture not amenable to ureteroureterostomy, where using an ileal interposition is not possible.

Ileal substitution of the ureter

Mochalova et al. reported two procedures under the heading "overpassing" anastomosis, probably referring to ileal ureter, one failed and the other successful as per their definition, at a follow-up of 20 and 25 years, respectively.[15]

Getahun et al. reported good outcomes (in terms of functional renal units) in 100% renal units (4/4) after an ileal replacement of the ureter at a median follow-up of 18 months.[17] The same group (Kumar et al.) later published their next decade experience with longer follow-up and found that 33.3% (2/6) renal units became nonfunctional based on an updated definition of nonfunction.[11]

Buccal Mucosa Augmentation of Upper Ureteric Structures

Kumar et al. reported this procedure in long segment upper ureteric strictures and found patent drainage and preserved renal function at 1 year follow-up (**Figs. 8.8 and 8.9**).[11] From this early report, it appears feasible; however, more data is needed before its outcome can be objectively assessed.

Bladder Augmentation

Kerr et al. reported outcomes of 12 patients with follow-up varying from 2 to 13 years. They report that trigone-sparing cystectomy gives better outcomes in terms of symptom improvement postoperatively. All 12 patients had good rehabilitation (symptom improvement) postoperatively. However, 58% (7/12) had infections, 16.6% (2/12) had new-onset or worsening hydronephrosis, and 33.3% (4/12) had metabolic abnormalities on follow-up. They do mention the possibility that some of these patients may have to be converted to an ileal conduit in order to salvage renal function.[3] A year later, an update discussed the follow-up of 14 patients; all but two had an incident-free follow-up. These two patients had a follow-up of 4 years and 13 years, respectively. The early complications within 2 years included fistula in one, retention followed by fistula in another and acidosis and uremia in two others. These early metabolic complications point toward low renal reserve in these patients. The late complications include new-onset hydronephrosis in one after 10 years, recurrent hypokalemia starting 2 years after surgery in one patient, episodes of pyelonephritis between 2 and 4 years of follow-up in two patients, recurrent

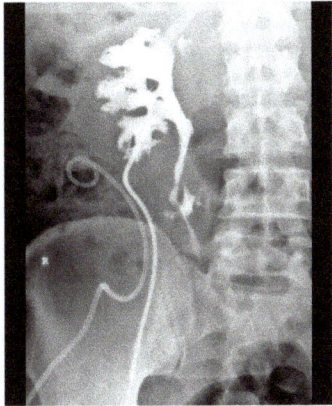

FIG. 8.8: Antegrade nephrostogram showing the right upper ureteric stricture and extravasation of the iodine radiocontrast.

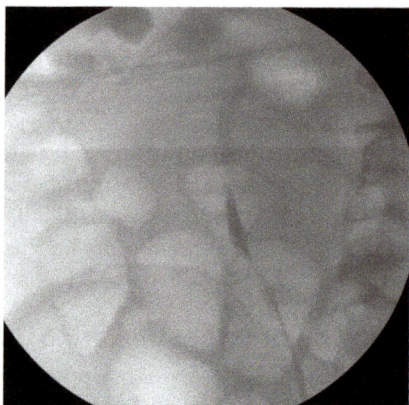

FIG. 8.9: The retrograde ureterogram of same renal unit as shown in Figure 8.8, status upper ureteric stricture repair with buccal mucosa and omental flap, showing the patent ureter, 6 months postoperatively.

TB after 2 years in one, enuresis starting after 9 and 11 years of follow-up in two patients, one patient requiring transurethral resection (TUR) for raised residual urine at 6 years of follow-up and another had an accidental death at 3 years' follow-up. Authors conclude that "in spite of intelligent diagnosis and management, these complications of cystoplasty for tuberculous contracture cloud the long-term prognosis in the majority of these patients; we still however, regard ileocystoplasty as a worthwhile operation."[14]

Mochalova et al. probably have the longest follow-up of augmentation cystoplasty using ileum and colon. They documented that the postoperative mortality was 4.4% in the first 15 days, 1.3% for the first year, 3.2% for 1–2 years, 2% for 2–5 years, 0.9% for 5–10 years, and 0.3% for 10–15 years. From 2–5 years, stenosis between the ureter and colon or colon and bladder was the main reason for mortality. Mortality in the subsequent years was due to chronic kidney disease.[15] This data points toward the fact that renal decompensation resulting in failure is the most important cause of ongoing mortality in this group of patients.

Getahun et al., in their 5-year retrospective analysis, reported poor outcomes in terms of renal function in 28.5 %(2/7) renal units following augmentation cystoplasty. None of the renal units undergoing ureteric reimplant with augmentation cystoplasty (four renal units) and ileal ureter with augmentation cystoplasty (three renal units) became nonfunctional as per the definition used in the study at 18 months of median follow-up.[17] Kumar et al. reported that 25% (1/4) renal units in the isolated augmentation cystoplasty group, 16% (3/18) renal units in the augmentation cystoplasty with ureteric reimplant group, 25% (2/8) renal units in the augmentation cystoplasty with bilateral ureteric implant group and none out of two in the ileal ureter with augmentation cystoplasty group became nonfunctional, as per the definition used in the study, at a mean follow-up of 61 months.[11]

Wagaskar et al. have reported poor outcomes of augmentation cystoplasty done for patients with nadir serum creatinine of 2–2.25 mg/dL (a serum creatinine of 2 mg/dL corresponds to an surface area standardized eGFR of 42 mL/min based on the CKD-EPI 2009 serum creatinine-based equation). Out of 5 patients, two required suprapubic continuous drainage and the other three required bilateral percutaneous nephrostomies for stabilization of renal function and prevention of recurrent urinary tract infections.[16] This experience suggests that the safe eGFR for offering augmentation is probably 60 mL/min/1.73 m². At the same time, such patients' disease may have evolving ureteric strictures, which may manifest with strictures at the reimplant site. This is the group in whom renal function was stabilized by percutaneous nephrostomies.

Another important complication noted in literature regarding augmentation cystoplasty for tubercular small capacity bladder is anastomotic stricture and diverticulum formation. Hemal et al. reported four cases of "diverticulization" and one case of spontaneous rupture due to anastomotic stricture out of the 80 patients their center had operated on.[12] They propose that thick fibrotic bladder with capacity <15–20 mL was one factor responsible for this complication; hence, they suggest offering orthotopic neobladder reconstruction in patients with small thick fibrotic bladder with capacity <20 mL, especially when associated with suprapubic pain and lower ureteric involvement.

From the above literature, it is clear that augmentation cystoplasty should be offered to appropriately selected and motivated patients. Augmentation cystoplasty does provide good symptomatic improvement. Even in appropriately selected patients, patient's motivation and regular follow-up by a dedicated urologist is of paramount importance. Long-term commitment on behalf of both the patient and the urologist, in order to prevent and manage complications that may impact renal function and hence overall survival is the key, as this is the most important outcome.

Orthotopic Substitution

Hemal et al. reported outcomes of four patients undergoing orthotopic neobladder (for tubercular small capacity bladders < 20 mL) with a mean follow-up duration of 38 months (22–54 months). They noted that one male patient required self-calibration for 3 months and required periodic dilatations. There was no symptomatic urinary tract infection or deterioration in renal function in these four patients.[12] Though not mentioned in the study, all long-term complications of augmentation cystoplasty are expected in this procedure as well, in addition to a higher incidence of stress incontinence.

Ileal Conduits

Getahun et al. reported good renal function in four patients undergoing diversion with an ileal conduit.[17] Kumar et al. reported 22.2% (4/18) renal units had final eGFR <15 mL/min at the last follow-up, after undergoing urinary diversion with ileal conduit.[11]

Wagaskar et al. have reported two patients with serum creatinine >2.5 mg/dL, who underwent short ileal conduit with night-time drainage. Their serum creatinine on follow-up was around 2.6 mg%. They feel that ileal conduits are preferable to augmentation cystoplasty in preserving renal function in the subgroup of patients with nadir serum creatinine >2 mg/dL.[16]

Urethroplasty

Mochalova et al. reported their experience of partially replacing urethra with a segment of ileum and two-third patients were reported to have successful outcomes at follow-up ranging from 10–20 years.[15] The diagnosis of a tubercular urethral stricture is mostly an exception rather than a rule. Once the appropriate diagnosis and medical treatment have been done, management should be like any other urethral stricture. Tubercular urethral involvement is one of the rare causes of failed urethroplasty and should be kept in mind. The authors have personal experience of one such case.

This chapter gives the brief short- and long-term outcomes of the various reconstructive procedures reported in literature for urinary TB. A few other important issues concerning reconstructive procedures are:

1. *What is the efficacy of reconstructive procedures as compared to long-term diversion in the form of double J stent or percutaneous nephrostomies in terms of renal unit function preservation?*
   Kumar et al. studied the baseline and final (involved) renal unit eGFR between the long-term diversion and reconstructive procedure groups. They found that reconstructive procedures are better at preserving baseline renal function as compared to long-term double J stenting or percutaneous nephrostomies.[11] The study was retrospective and accepts and details the inherent bias in patient selection in that the better functioning renal units were subjected to reconstructive procedures. The authors suggest that whenever feasible reconstruction should be offered in preference to long-term diversion, even if that means referring the patient to a high-volume center which is comfortable in doing such procedures.

2. *What is the comparative efficacy of various reconstructive procedures?*
   Lower tract renal drainage procedures have better outcomes in terms of renal unit function preservation as compared to upper tract drainage procedures.[11] This means we need to find better alternatives to the present surgical procedures available for upper tract drainage. This finding may also suggest that renal units requiring upper tract reconstruction are more damaged kidneys. This question needs to be addressed by properly planned prospective studies.

3. *Is renal unit function preservation by reconstructive procedures a function of time?*
   Reconstructive surgical procedures in addition to immediate complications have a long-term time-dependent failure rate in terms of renal function which is not well documented in literature but suggested by at least one retrospective study.[11] This makes the case for their longer follow-up, especially in cases where backup reconstruction is feasible. The long-term, time-dependent failure of the reconstructive surgery supports the hypothesis that the tissue used for the reconstruction has a half-life. Hence, better quality of tissue used for reconstruction (in terms of vascularity, innervation, and absence of pathology) ensures better long-term outcomes.

4. *What is the most important factor predicting successful outcome in patients with urinary TB?*
   The most important factor for renal function preservation is the baseline renal function, irrespective of the type of reconstruction procedure used.[11] This suggests that earlier diagnosis would ensure better outcomes. Future improvements in diagnostics may result in earlier diagnosis; however, as genitourinary physicians and surgeons, it is our responsibility to be aware of the various presentations of this pathology which is instrumental to early diagnosis and management.

LIMITATIONS OF THE PRESENT LITERATURE

Absence of objective documentation of involved renal unit function pre- and postoperatively hampers the assessment of surgical outcomes, especially if a normal functioning opposite kidney is present and the reconstruction did not affect the contralateral kidney. In cases of bladder reconstruction, global renal function is the outcome of interest and easier to assess and document. For the sake of future research, single renal unit eGFR would be the preferred assessment tool for defining outcomes in addition to symptom improvement assessment.

Secondly, the failure to report retrospective data using standardized tools, such as Kaplan–Meier survival estimator, makes it difficult to compare the outcomes of different centers.

Thirdly, there is a lack of prospective long-term studies on the topic. Renal unit loss is less likely to be symptomatic, especially if the process has been insidious and the opposite renal unit function is normal. Hence, there is a high likelihood that such patients would never seek medical assistance. This would lead to overestimation of success based on renal unit function assessment, especially in retrospective series. Even in prospective series where only symptomatic patients were followed up and split renal function assessment was not carried out at follow-up, overestimation of successful outcomes is a possibility. Prospective data, with longer follow-up using objective outcome parameter assessment, would give a clearer picture of the outcomes of these surgical procedures in the future.

Future research aiming to resolve the above-mentioned limitations would be the way forward.

REFERENCES

1. Harris RI, Kerr WK, Coulthard HS. Renal tuberculosis: Long-term review of cases followed-up from twenty to thirty-five years. Br J Surg. 1960;47(205):539-42.
2. Gow JG. Genitourinary tuberculosis: A study of short course regimens. J Urol. 1976;115(6):707-11.
3. Kerr WK, Gale GL, Peterson KSS. Reconstructive surgery for genitourinary tuberculosis. J Urol. 1969;101(3):254-66.
4. Barrie HJ, Kerr WK, Gale GL. The Incidence and Pathogenesis of tuberculous strictures of the renal pyelus. J Urol. 1967;98(5):584-9.
5. Levey AS, de Jong PE, Coresh J, El Nahas M, Astor BC, Matsushita K, et al. The definition, classification, and prognosis of chronic kidney disease: a KDIGO Controversies Conference report. Kidney Int. 2011;80(1):17-28.
6. Gow JG. Genitourinary Tuberculosis: A 7-Year Review. Br J Urol. 1979;51(4):239-44.
7. Flechner SM, Gow JG. Role of nephrectomy in the treatment of non-functioning or very poorly functioning unilateral tuberculous kidney. J Urol. 1980;123(6):822-5.
8. Bloom S, Wechsler H, Lattimer JK. Results of a long-term study of non-functioning tuberculous kidneys. J Urol. 1970;104(5):654-7.
9. Krishnamoorthy S, Gopalakrishnan G. Surgical management of renal tuberculosis. Indian J Urol. 2008;24(3):369.
10. Viswaroop B, Gopalakrishnan G, Nath V, Kekre NS. Role of imaging in predicting salvageability of kidneys in urinary tract tuberculosis. J Pak Med Assoc. 2006;56(12):587-90.
11. Kumar A, Dangi AD, Mukha RP, Panda A, Jeychandraberry C, Kumar S, et al. Can kidneys be saved in patients with urinary tuberculosis? A study in the era of modern chemotherapy and surgical armamentarium. Int J Urol. 2019;26(5):551-7.
12. Hemal AK, Aron M. Orthotopic neobladder in management of tubercular thimble bladders: initial experience and long-term results. Urology. 1999;53(2):298-301.
13. Singh P, Bansal A, Sekhon V, Nunia S, Ansari MS. Can baseline serum creatinine and e-GFR predict renal function outcome after augmentation cystoplasty in children? Int Braz J Urol. 2018;44(1):156-62.
14. Kerr WK, Gale GL, Struthers NW, Peterson KSS, Coulthard HS, Greatrex GE, et al. Prognosis in reconstructive surgery for urinary tuberculosis. Br J Urol. 1970;42(6):672-8.
15. Mochalova TP, Starikov IY. Reconstructive surgery for treatment of urogenital tuberculosis: 30 years of observation. World J Surg. 1997;21(5):511-5.
16. Wagaskar VG, Chirmade RA, Baheti VH, Tanwar HV, Patwardhan SK, Gopalakrishnan G. Urinary tuberculosis with renal failure: challenges in management. J Clin Diagn Res. 2016;10(1):PC01-3.
17. Getahun GM, Prasad S, Chako N, Goplakrishnan G. Outcomes of reconstructive surgery of tuberculosis affecting the ureter and bladder. East Cent Afr J Surg. 2009;14(2):85-88–88.

CHAPTER 9

Interesting Cases

Ganesh Gopalakrishnan, Sujata Patwardhan, Ajit Sawant, Umesh Shelke

CASE 1

A 52-year-old male presented with persistent cough, decreased appetite, and weight loss. There was no history of any comorbid illness.

Examination findings were normal.

Hematological investigations revealed elevated ESR, decreased hemoglobin (9.2 g/dL) with raised serum creatinine (2.4 mg/dL).

Urinalysis revealed plenty of pus cells. On culture, *Escherichia coli* was grown.

Initial radiological evaluation with USG revealed gross right hydronephrosis.

CT-KUB plain showed bulky right kidney with caliectasis with perinephric fat stranding and perinephric collection extending into psoas muscle. There were multiple parenchymal calcification areas with one inferior calyceal stone. Large upper ureteric stone was seen with ureteric wall thickening. Left kidney was normal except for a mid pole simple cyst (**Figs. 1A to E**).

PCN was done which drained thick pus.

EC scan was done which revealed nonfunctioning right kidney.

Right nephrectomy was done. Intraoperative injury occurred to second portion of duodenum due to dense perinephric adhesions. Duodenal repair was done.

On taking cuts of specimen, there were multiple dilated calyces with thick pultaceous material inside.

Histopathological examination revealed caseous necrotizing granulomatous inflammation due to tuberculosis.

Patient was started on AKT postoperatively.

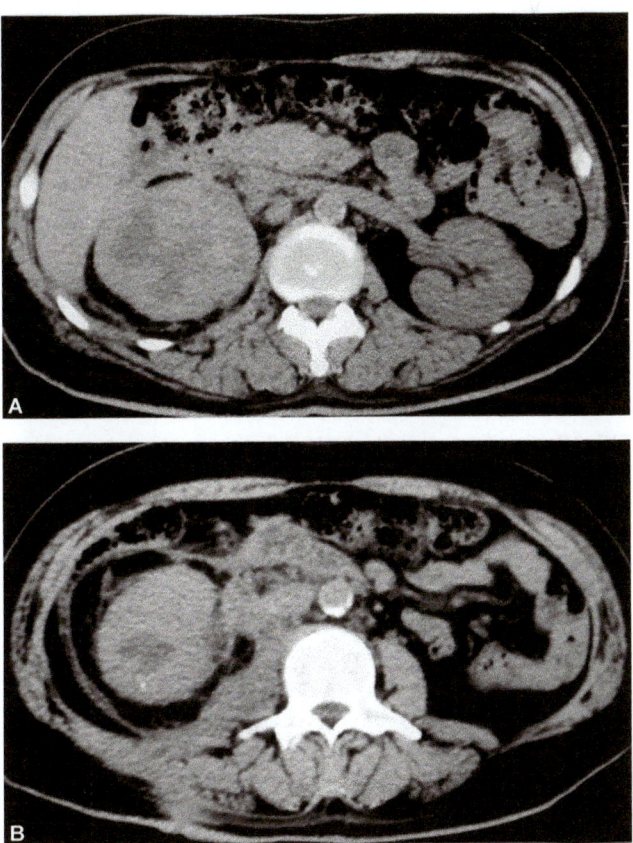

FIGS. 1A AND B: Developing abscess in medulla and cortex in multiple areas.

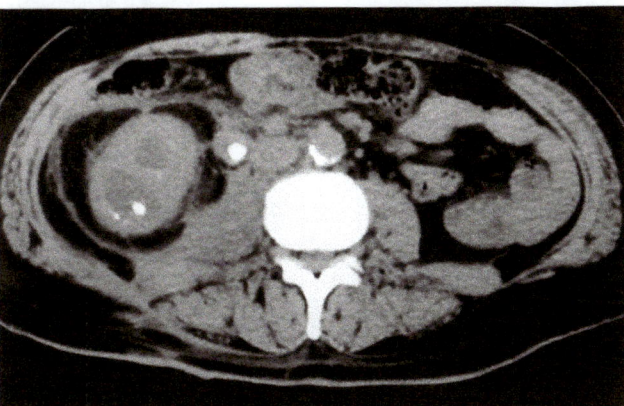

FIG. 1C: Calcification in the wall of the abscess with perinephric fat stranding, involvement of psoas, and calculus in ureter.

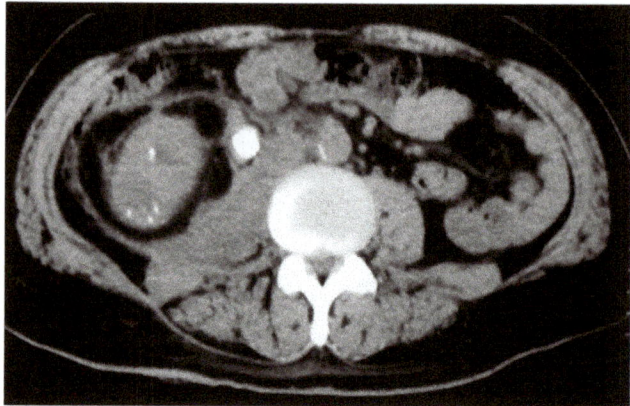

FIG. 1D: Calcification in the wall of the abscess with perinephric fat stranding, involvement of psoas, and calculus in ureter with collection beyond Gerota's fascia.

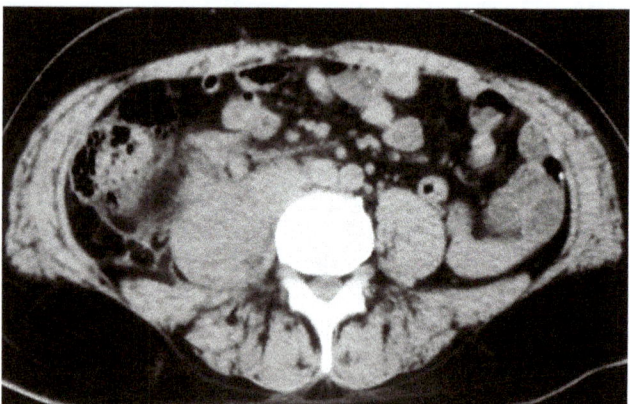

FIG. 1E: Psoas abscess.

CASE 2

An 18-year-old thin built female patient presented with multiple episodes of high-grade fever with chills within a span of 2 weeks with decreased appetite, nausea, and vomiting.

On examination, there was tenderness in left lumbar region and renal angle.

Hematological investigations revealed leukocytosis (25,000/mm^3) with raised serum creatinine (1.8 mg/dL).

Ultrasonogram revealed grossly dilated left kidney with thick moving internal echoes in dilated calyces with multiple renal abscesses.

CT scan done showed left enlarged kidney with dilated calyces with infundibular stenosis suggestive of phantom calyces. There was left hydronephrosis and hydroureter with thickened ureteric wall (**Figs. 2A to E**) with narrowing at lower ureter. There were multiple calcification foci in ureteric wall and renal parenchyma.

There was large perinephric abscess extending into psoas muscle (**Figs. 2F to J**).

Left PCN was done. There was thick pus which was sent for evaluation. It was positive for TB-PCR and TB-MGIT. Patient was started on Category 1 AKT.

Six months after completion of AKT, patient improved clinically. There were no episodes of pyelonephritis. Patient gained weight with improved appetite.

PCN output about 1.2 L/day. Serum creatinine came to nadir of 1.5 mg/dL.

Left ureteric reimplantation with psoas hitch was done for left lower ureteric stricture.

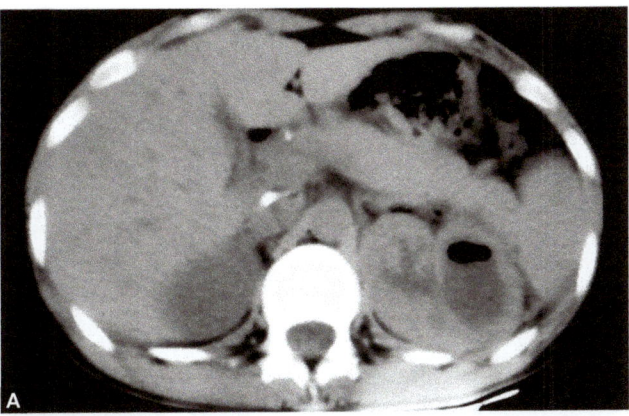

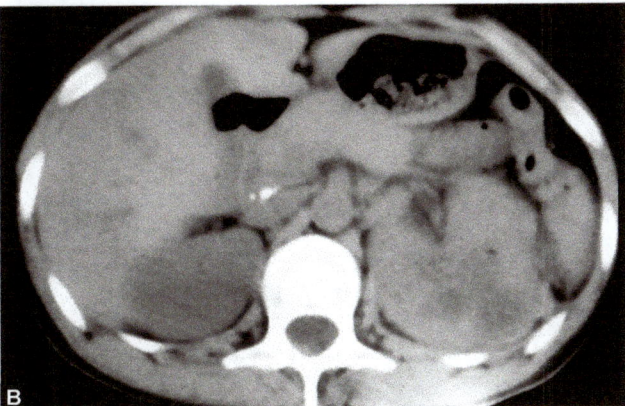

FIGS. 2A AND B: Multiple abscess in medulla with air foci.

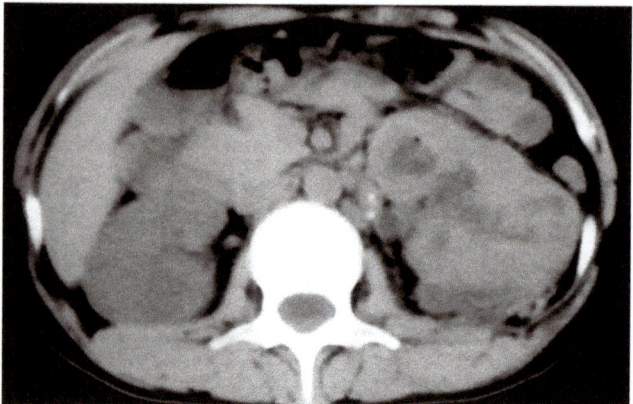

FIG. 2C: Multiple abscess in medulla with perirenal extension and thickened ureter.

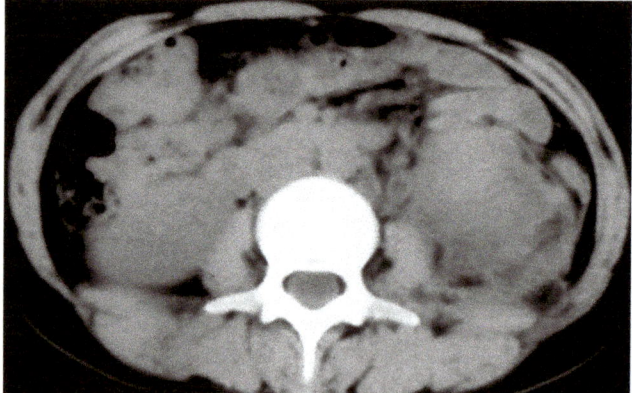

FIG. 2D: Involvement of the psoas and adjacent abdominal wall.

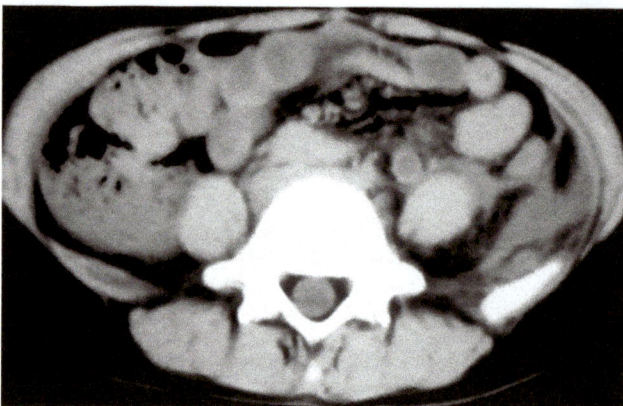

FIG. 2E: Thickened ureter.

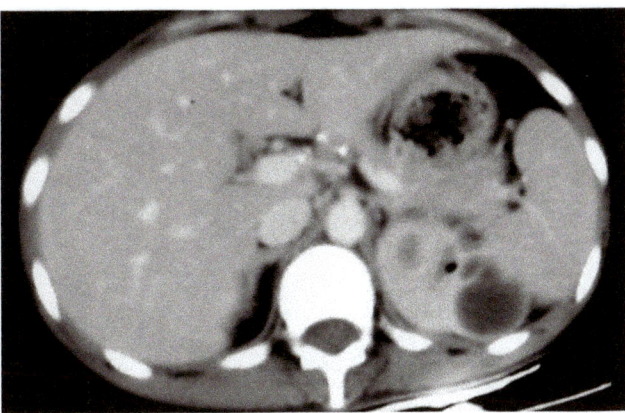

FIG. 2F: Developing abscess.

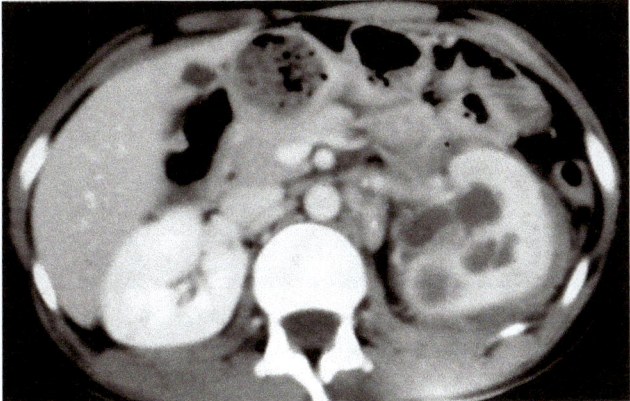

FIG. 2G: Thick-walled abscess in the cortex with perirenal fat stranding.

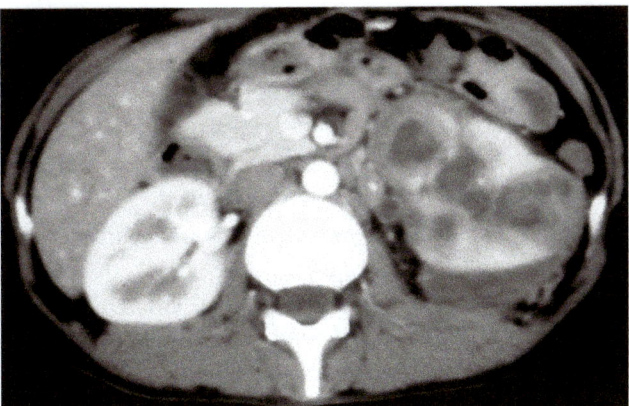

FIG. 2H: Renal abscess and ureteric wall calcification and thickening.

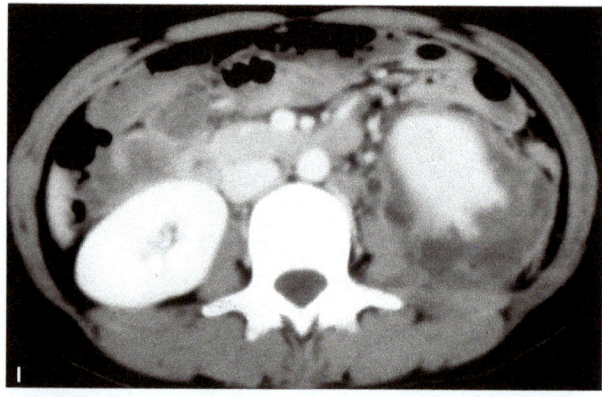

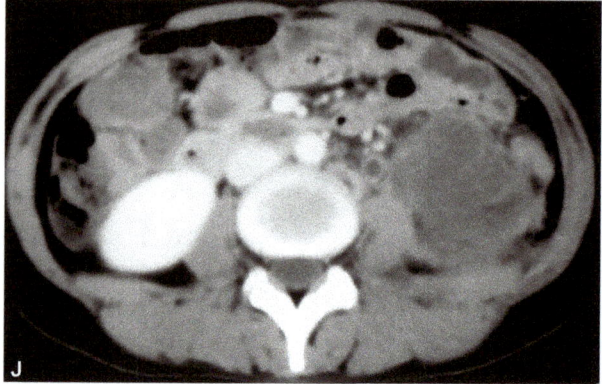

FIGS. 2I AND J: Perirenal extension of the abscess involving psoas and posterior abdominal wall.

CASE 3

A 48-year-old male presented with poor stream of urine, straining during micturition, left flank pain, decreased appetite, and nausea and vomiting. Examination findings were normal, except for mild tenderness in left flank.

Hematological investigations: Hb: 7.2, WBC: 15,300/mm^3, and serum creatinine: 3.2 mg/dL which decreased to 2 mg% after few weeks of diversion.

On ultrasonogram, there was bilateral hydronephrosis and hydroureter till VUJ.

CT scan revealed small, grossly hydronephrotic right kidney with dilated calyces and contracted pelvis with calcification at lower pole with thinned parenchyma. Left kidney also was grossly hydronephrotic with thickened ureter and perirenal abscess extending into psoas muscle with small capacity, thick-walled bladder (**Figs. 3A to G**).

Left PCN was done. Patient's all urine output was through left PCN with no output per urethrally (**Fig. 3H**).

RGU was done to evaluate urethra. There was stricture in the bulbar segment.

PCN fluid sent for evaluation was positive for TB-PCR.

Patient was started on Category 1 AKT.

After completion of AKT, patient underwent permanent perineal urethrostomy with augmentation ileocystoplasty with right nephrectomy and left ureteric reimplantation.

HPR of the distal urethra revealed evidence of chronic granulomatous inflammation suggestive of tuberculosis etiology.

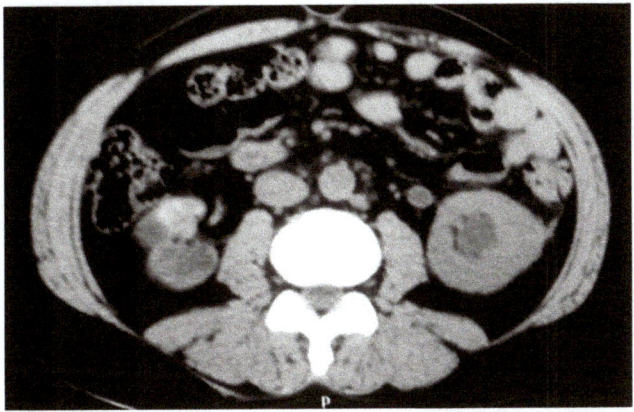

FIG. 3A: Calcification in the right lower pole with multiple abscesses with dilated left ureter.

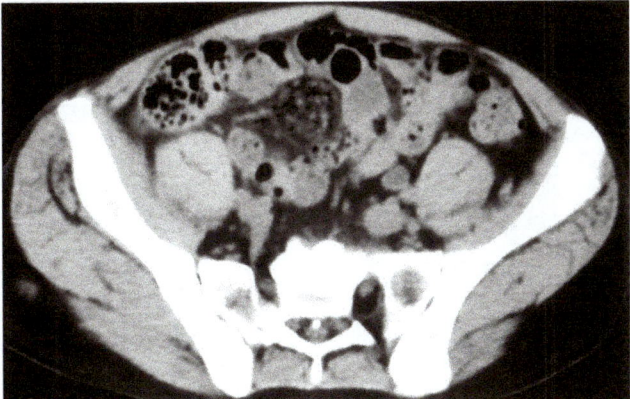

FIG. 3B: Right psoas abscess.

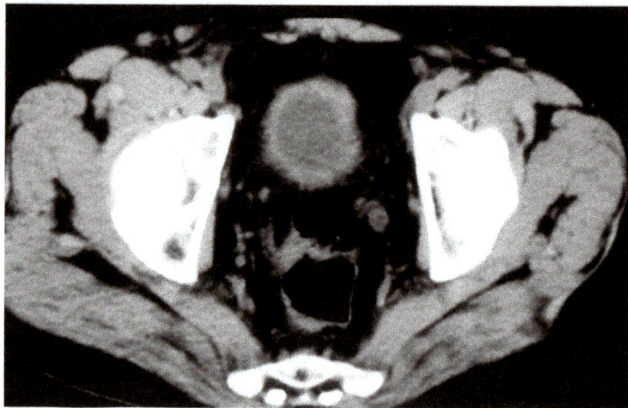

FIG. 3C: Thickened bladder.

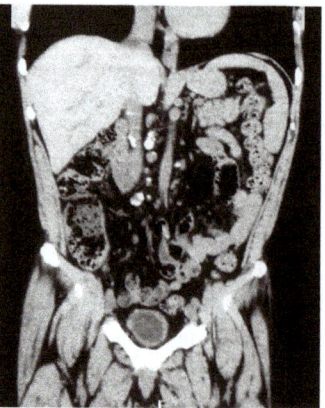

FIG. 3D: Calcification in the retroperitoneal lymph nodes, kidney, and thickened bladder.

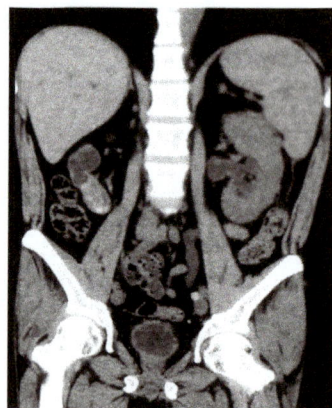

FIG. 3E: Calcified lower pole of right kidney.

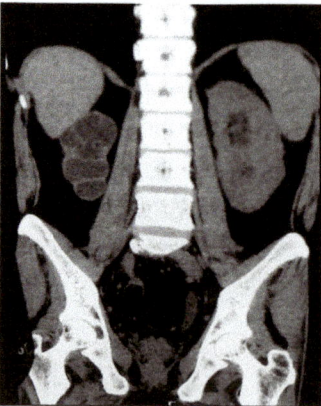

FIG. 3F: Shrunken, nonfunctioning right kidney.

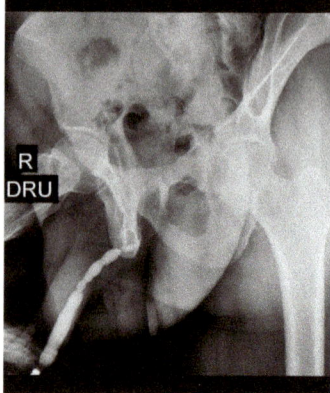

FIG. 3G: DRU with multiple strictures in the bulbar urethra.

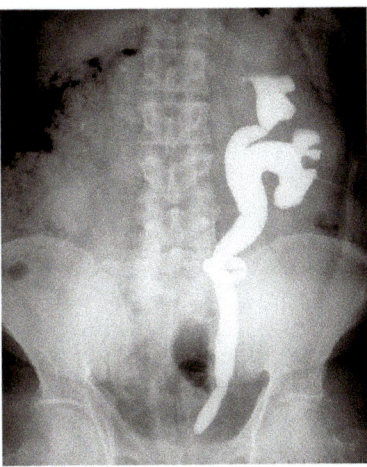

(PCN-O: percutaneous nephrostomy-obstruction)
FIG. 3H: PCN-O-gram with left lower ureteric stricture.

CASE 4

A 62-year-old male patient presented with bilateral flank pain, low-grade fever, decreased appetite, nausea, and vomiting since 2–3 months. There was h/o spine tuberculosis 20 years back for which patient had received treatment but details of treatment were not available (**Fig. 4A**). Physical examination was normal.

On hematological examination: Hb: 8.2 g/dL, Creatinine: 3.2 mg/dL.

Urinalysis revealed plenty of pus cells.

USG (done at the time of AKI episode) revealed bilateral hydronephrosis and hydroureter with left renal calculi.

Six months' old IVP showed bilateral hydronephrosis and hydroureter with left renal calculi with narrowing in bilateral lower ureter with small capacity bladder (**Figs. 4B and C**).

Chest X-ray showed egg shell calcifications in hilar and para tracheal group of lymphnodes (**Fig. 4D**).

Fresh CT KUB plain revealed bilateral hydronephrosis and hydroureter with left renal calculi. There was left lower ureteric wall thickening with calcification in the wall. Bladder wall was thickened and appeared small in capacity (**Figs. 4E and F**).

Bilateral PCN were inserted. Bilateral PCN fluid samples were sent for evaluation. Report was positive for TB-MGIT and TB-PCR. Patient was started on AKT.

After 2 months of AKT and PCN drainage, serum creatinine came down to 2.7 as nadir level. Left PCNL was done to clear the stone.

MCU revealed small capacity bladder with right-sided grade 4 reflux.

Short segment ileal conduit diversion with bilateral ileoureteral anastomosis was done in this patient.

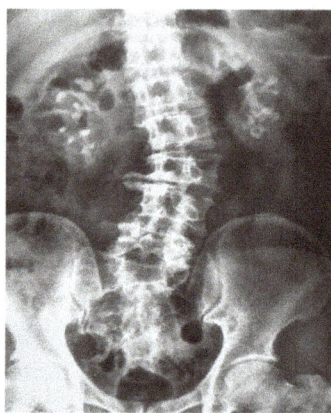

FIG. 4A: Old healed Pott's spine with left renal calcification.

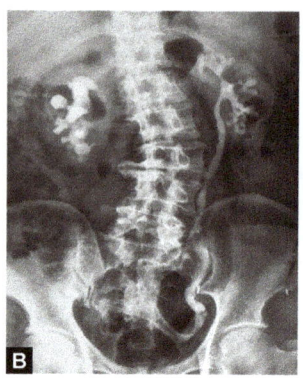
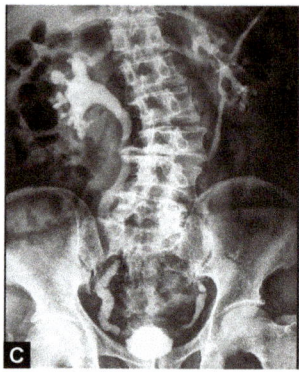
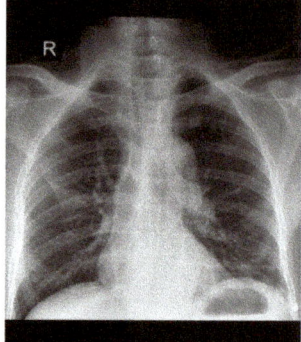

FIGS. 4B AND C: Thick-walled calyces, distorted pelvicalyceal system with calcification.

FIG. 4D: Eggshell calcification in paratracheal and hilar lymph nodes.

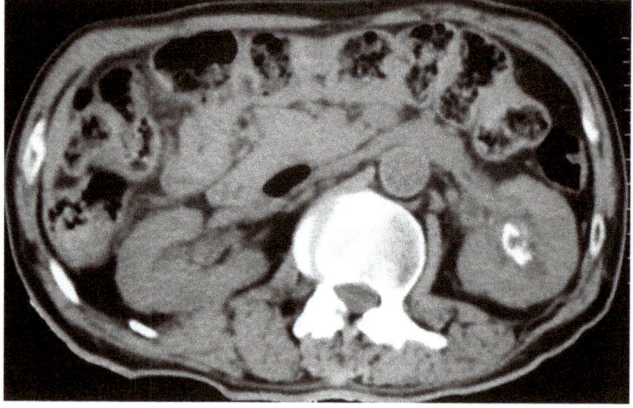

FIG. 4E: CT films showing left renal parenchymal calcification.

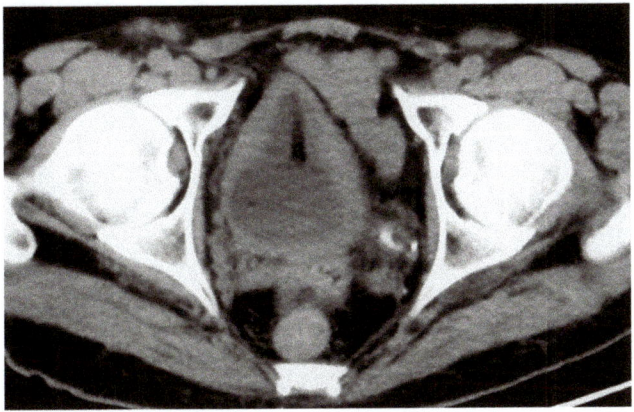

FIG. 4F: Thick-walled bladder with left ureteric wall calcification.

CASE 5

A 42-year-old male patient presented with increased frequency, urgency, nocturia, and dysuria since last 4 years. Patient also had bilateral flank pain since 1 year. He had dry ejaculation during intercourse with occasional hematospermia.

On examination, there were bilateral enlarged testis and epididymis, and hard consistency at some areas with bilateral thickened spermatic cord.

Hematological investigations revealed low hemoglobin (7.6 g/dL) and serum creatinine 1.7 mg/dL.

Urinalysis revealed plenty of pus cells. Initial culture was positive for *Escherichia coli*.

Ultrasonogram was done which showed moderate hydronephrosis in right kidney with shrunken left kidney.

Plain CT was done. There was hydronephrosis and hydroureter on right side with narrowing at VUJ. Left kidney was shrunken, small with parenchymal calcifications in it. Urinary bladder was small and contracted with thickened walls (**Figs. 5A to F**).

Initially right PCN was done and urine was sent for urinalysis. It was positive for urine AFB.

Patient was started on Category 1 AKT.

After completion of AKT, left-sided nephrectomy and augmentation ileocystoplasty with right ureteric reimplantation was done.

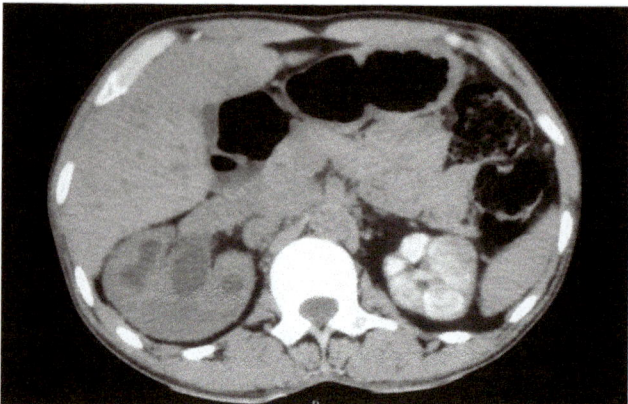

FIG. 5A: Right hydronephrosis with left parenchymal calcification and calcification in the wall of tuberculoma.

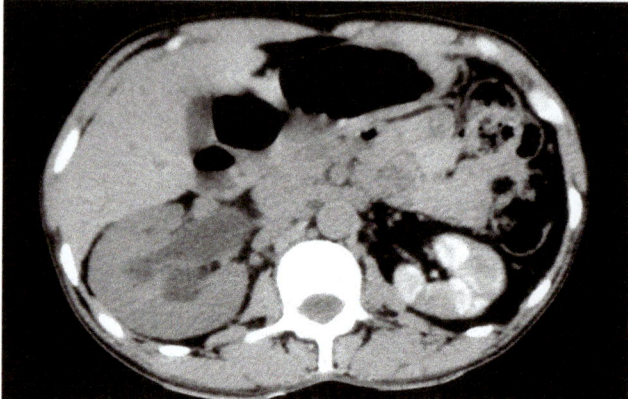

FIG. 5B: Right kidney with unequally dilated calyces with left parenchymal calcification and calcification in the wall of tuberculoma.

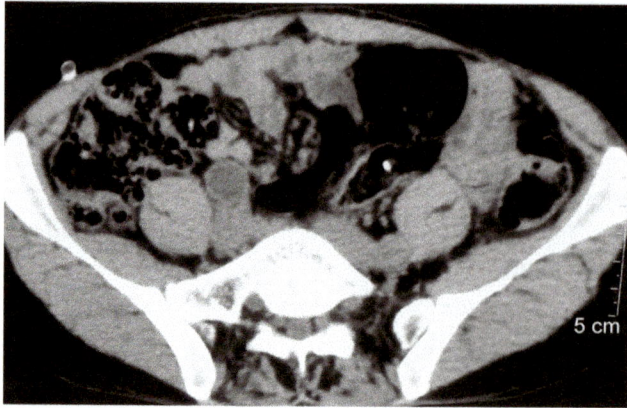

FIG. 5C: Dilated right ureter with thick walls.

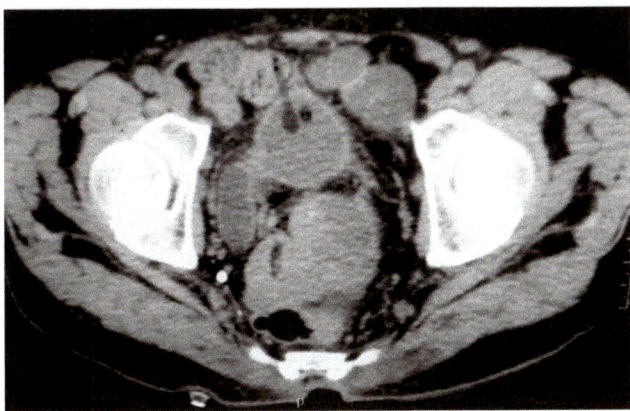

FIG. 5D: Stricture at the right vesicoureteric junction.

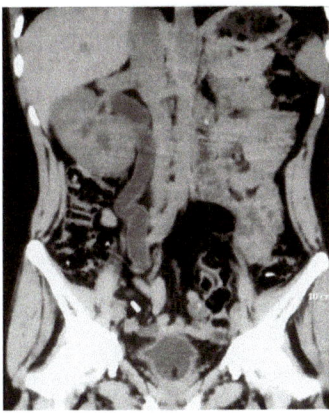

FIG. 5E: Hypodense areas in right renal parenchyma with left shrunken kidney with dilated thickened right ureter.

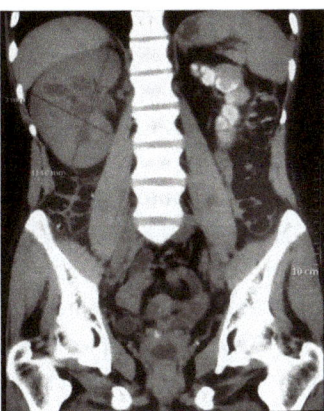

FIG. 5F: Right renal parenchyma showing hypodense areas with distorted calyces and left putty kidney.

CASE 6

A 21-year-old male presented with right flank pain, decreased appetite, nausea, vomiting, and intermittent episodes of high-grade fever with chills since few days. Patient was a k/c/o extrahepatic portal hypertension with hypersplenism.

Examination revealed tenderness in right flank with localized guarding.

Hematological investigations revealed 7.2 g/dL hemoglobin, 1.2 mg/dL serum creatinine. Platelet and leukocyte counts were 52,000 and 4,200/mm^3, respectively.

Urinalysis showed plenty of pus cells.

On ultrasonogram, there was grossly hydronephrotic right kidney with internal moving echoes. There was perinephric collection tracking along psoas muscle on right side. Left kidney was normal.

PCN was done in emergency for pyonephrosis and pigtail catheter insertion was done for perinephric and psoas abscesses.

Pus was positive for AFB on smear and culture.

On CT, right kidney was grossly hydronephrotic with dilated calyces. There was extension of the abscess into psoas muscle. There was upper ureteric calculus, calculus in inferior calyx, and parenchymal calcifications. Ureter was dilated and thickened proximal to stone. PCN drained 150 mL of pus and gradually PCN output decreased to nil (**Figs. 6A to F**).

EC scan was s/o nonfunctioning right kidney.

After completion of intensive phase of AKT, right nephrectomy was done. Histopathology was s/o multiple caseating granulomatous inflammation involving entire kidney.

After 2 years, patient presented with continuous minimal drainage of pus through prior drain site scar.

Pus was negative for AFB and TB MGIT but it failed to heal even on antibiotic course. ESR was 55 mm/h.

Tract was cannulated. Repeat CT was done.

CT was s/o fistulous tract extending from skin to psoas muscle and ureter with calcification areas along the tract (**Figs. 6A to F**).

Patient underwent fistula tract excision.

Histopathology was s/o fibrosis and multiple granulomas in the tract.

Ideally, the tissue should have been sent for culture to detect any resistance. Patient was started on Category 1 AQKT again for 6 months. He was asymptomatic.

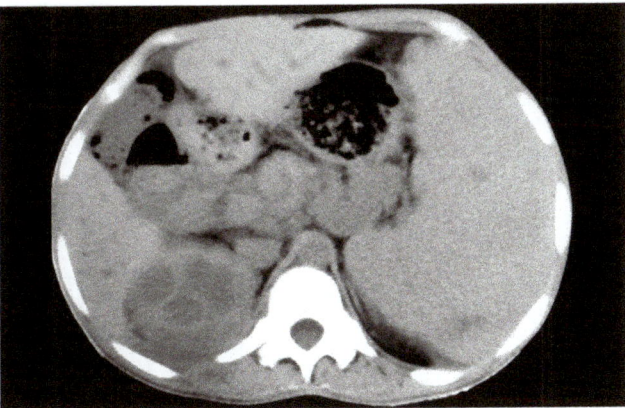

(PCS: pelvicalyceal system)
FIG. 6A: Right renal parenchyma showing multiple hypodensities with distorted PCS.

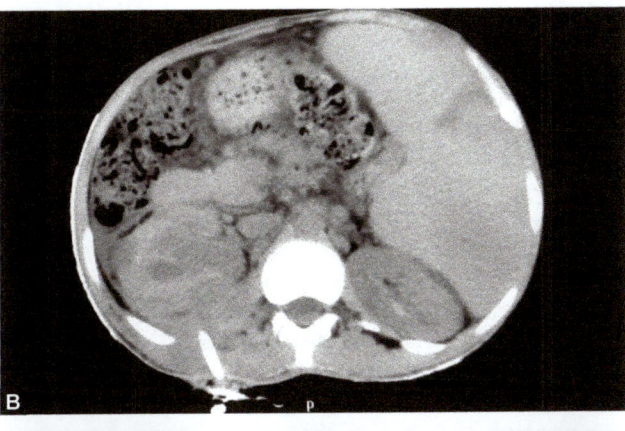

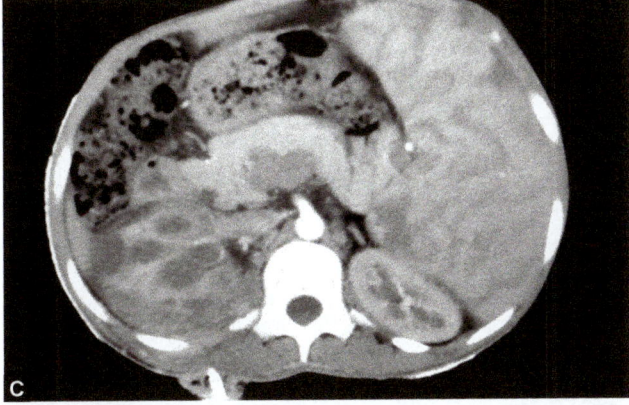

FIGS. 6B AND C: Right renal abscess with extension into perirenal space and the psoas muscle.

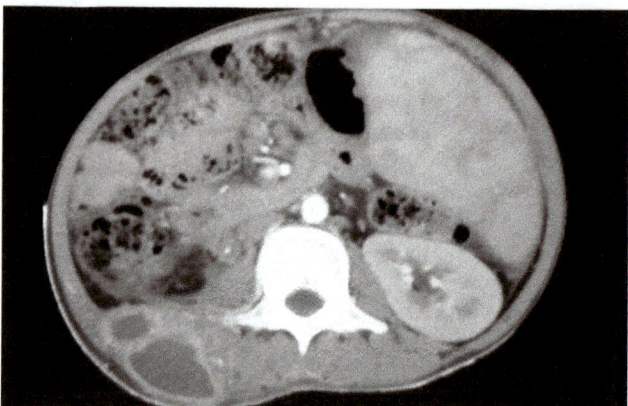

FIG. 6D: Right thick-walled, dilated ureter with wall calcification.

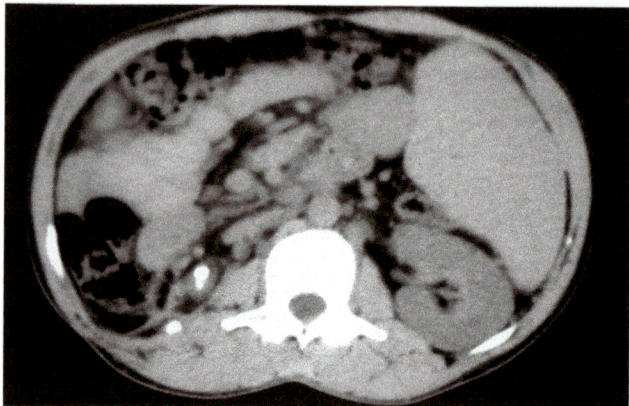

FIG. 6E: Contrast in the sinus tract showing thick-walled sinus tract with calcification.

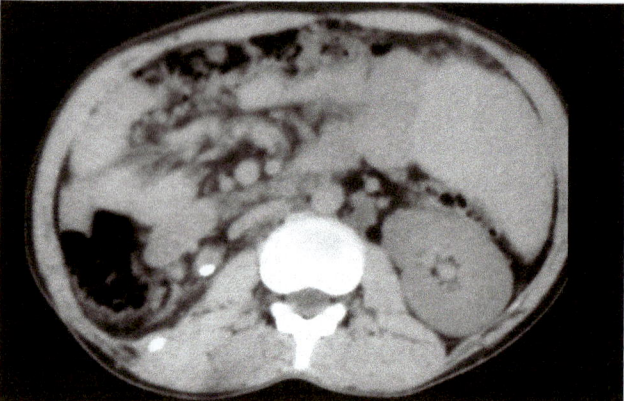

FIG. 6F: Contrast in the sinus tract showing thick-walled sinus tract with calcification.

CASE 7

A 54-year-old male presented with c/o increased frequency of diurnal and nocturnal, urgency, urge incontinence, and dysuria since 4 years. Patient was evaluated for same and was diagnosed to have small capacity bladder for which augmentation cystoplasty was done 2 years back.

Patient at the age of 35 years was diagnosed to have pulmonary tuberculosis for which AKT course was completed. Then patient developed repeated episodes of dizziness, fainting episodes, and dark pigmentation of skin for which patient was evaluated and found to have adrenal insufficiency secondary to adrenal tuberculosis. Patient again received course of AKT and was started on steroids and mineralocorticoid supplementation.

On examination, patient had dark pigmented skin. Rest examination was normal.

On hematological investigations, Hb was 9.2 g/dL and serum creatinine was 2.6 mg/dL.

On urinalysis, there were plenty of pus cells.

USG revealed bilateral hydronephrosis and hydroureter with small capacity bladder.

On CT, there was bilateral entire hydronephrosis and hydroureter with small capacity bladder with thickened, irregular bladder wall (**Figs. 7A and B**).

Cystogram study revealed small capacity bladder with irregular walls with bilateral grade II passive reflux (**Fig. 7C**).

Patient underwent ileal conduit diversion for the same.

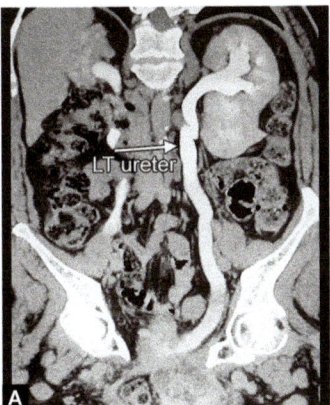 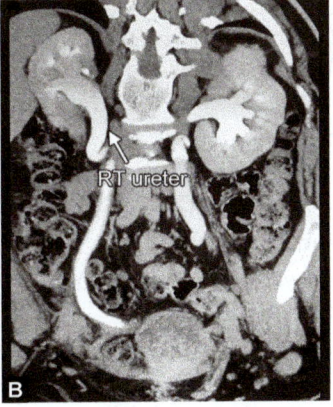

FIGS. 7A AND B: Bilateral hydroureteronephrosis with vesicoureteric junction obstruction.

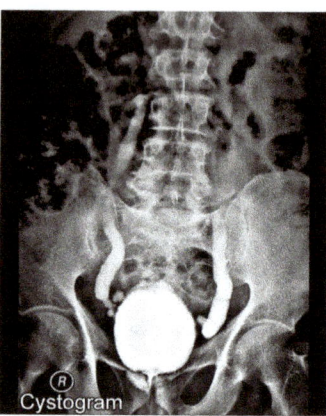

FIG. 7C: Micturating cystogram showing bilateral passive vesicoureteric reflux with small capacity bladder and bladder diverticulum with bilateral narrowing at vesicoureteric junction.

CASE 8

A 36-year-old female presented with increased frequency of diurnal and nocturnal, urgency, and urge incontinence since 7 months. Patient was diagnosed to have repeated UTI for which patient received antibiotics courses, only to cause partial symptomatic relief. Patient also started having left flank pain since last 4 months of dull aching and fever with chills since 1 month.

She also had primary infertility.

Examination findings were normal.

On hematology examination, Hb: 8.4 g/dL, WBC: 12,600/mm^3, serum creatinine: 1.6 mg/dL, and ESR: 60 mm/h.

On USG, there was left hydronephrosis, entire moderate hydroureter, and small capacity thick-walled bladder.

On CT, there was entire left HNHU with narrowing at lower ureter and small capacity bladder. Ureteric wall was thickened. There were multiple left renal parenchymal calcifications seen (**Figs. 8A to D**).

MCU was done which revealed small capacity bladder with bilateral high grade reflux with left lower ureteric stricture (**Fig. 8E**).

Left PCN was inserted and fluid was sent for R/M, AFB, culture and sensitivity.

It was positive for urine AFB smear and culture.

Patient was started on Category 1 AKT.

Antegrade dye study from left PCN revealed left lower ureteric stricture with unhealthy lower ureter (**Figs. 8F and G**).

Patient underwent augmentation cystoplasty with left ureteric reimplant in bowel segment.

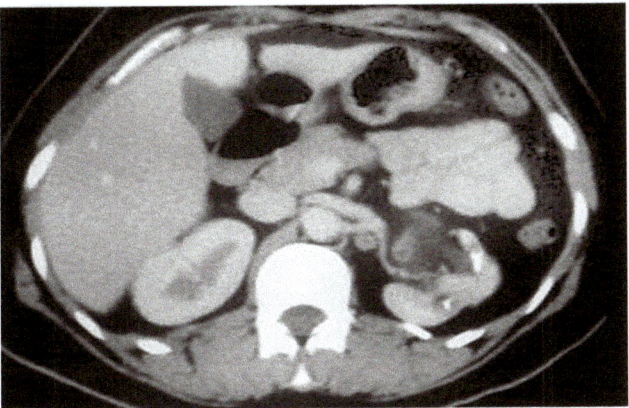

FIG. 8A: Left kidney showing parenchymal calcification with distorted calyces.

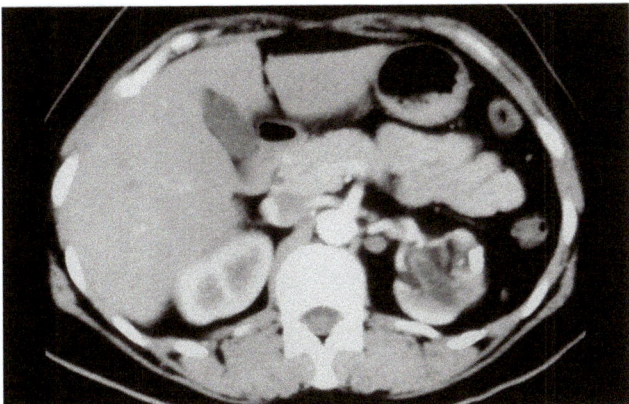

FIG. 8B: Left kidney showing distorted pelvicalyceal system with parenchymal calcification.

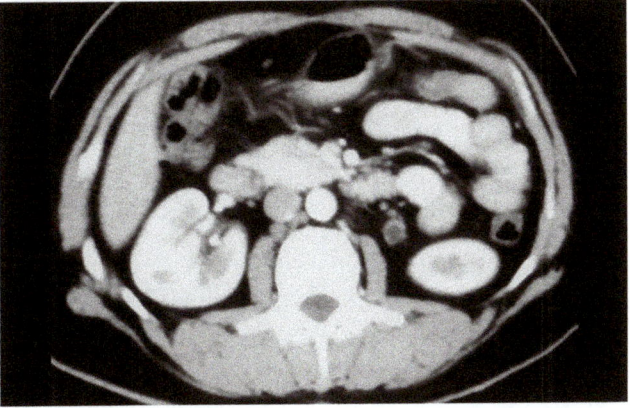

FIG. 8C: Left ureteric dilatation with wall thickening.

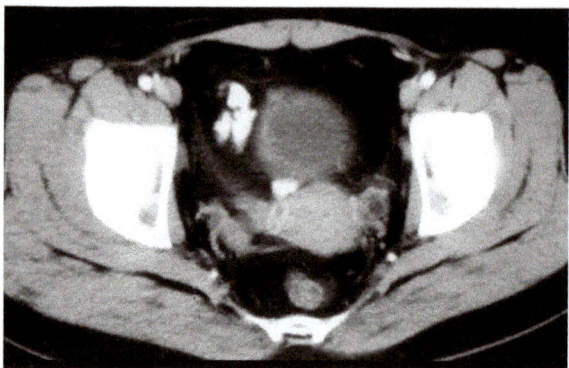

FIG. 8D: Thickened wall of bladder and left lower ureter present.

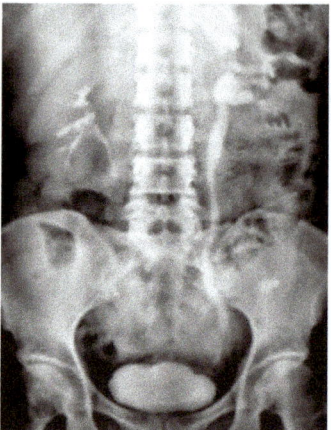

FIG. 8E: Micturating cystourethrogram showing bilateral vesico-ureteric reflux with left lower ureteric stricture.

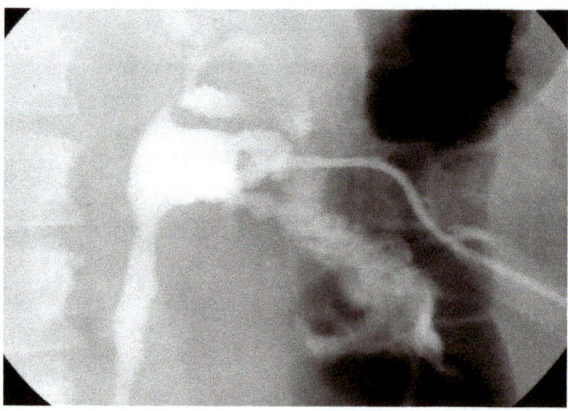

(PCN-O: percutaneous nephrostomy-obstruction)
FIG. 8F: PCN-O gram showing infundibular narrowing and irregular dilated calyces.

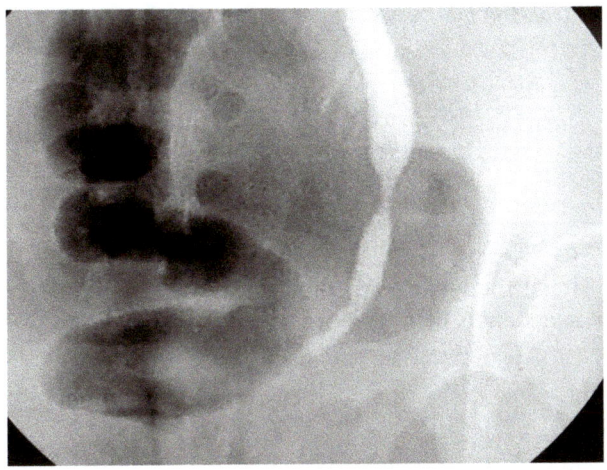

(PCN-O: percutaneous nephrostomy-obstruction)

FIG. 8G: PCN-O gram showing multiple left ureteric stricture in lower one third and vesicoureteric junction stricture.

CASE 9

A 25-year-old married female presented with h/o urinary frequency, dysuria with urgency and h/o passage of blood clots since 1 month. Patient underwent cystoscopy and cold cup biopsy elsewhere and histopathology reported as s/o granulomatous cystitis and tuberculosis.

Patient started on Category 1 AKT for 9 months.

Three months after initiation of AKT, patient presented with AKI and serum creatinine of 9.3 mg% and BUN: 90. Patient received one cycle of hemodialysis.

Plain CT KUB s/o bilateral hydroureteronephrosis for which B/L PCN insertion and creatinine decreased to 1.6 mg%.

Subsequently diagnosed to have small capacity bladder on MCU and reduced left renal function on DMSA.

Obstetric history: P2L1A1.

No h/o menstrual irregularities.

No past h/o pulmonary Koch's or Koch's contact.

General and systemic examination: NAD.

Investigations

Urine R/M: 6–8 pus cells/hpf; 38–40 RBCs/hpf.

Urine C/S: *Pseudomonas aeruginosa*.

Urine R/M (16/03/2016): 3–4 pus cells/hpf; 1–2 RBCs/hpf.
Urine C/S (17/03/2016): *Escherichia coli*.
Hb: 10.2 g%; TLC: 7,900/cmm.

Date	9/02/15	9/05/15	16/05/15	16/03/16	11/04/16
Serum creatinine	1.3	9.3	1.6 (after B/L PCN)	2.7	2.2
BUN		90.0		35	27

LFT and serum electrolytes: Normal.

CT urography: Bilateral moderate hydronephrosis and hydroureter with diffuse and irregular thickening of urinary bladder (**Figs. 9A and B**).

MCU: Left-grade III VUR with small capacity bladder (**Fig. 9C**).

PCN-O gram: Right—e/o contrast hold up at lower ureter (cutoff) s/o lower ureteric stricture (**Fig. 9D**).

Left contrast not entering into the ureter.

Urine AFB: Negative.

TB MGIT: No growth.

Urodynamic study: Unstable filling phase with reduced compliance.

DMSA renogram: Left K (34.83%); right K (65.17%).

Patient underwent augmentation ileocystoplasty with right ureteric reimplantation.

EC renogram after surgery:

	Left kidney	Right kidney
Differential function (%)	16.54	83.46
ERPF (mL/min)	30.15	152.19

Serum creatinine: 2.0 mg%.
BUN: 21.4 mg%.
Left nephrectomy: Done.
HPR: Granulomatous infection suggestive of tuberculosis.

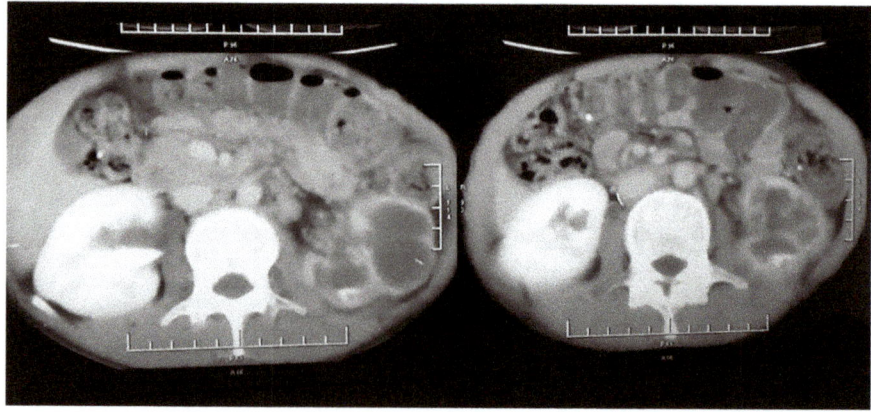

FIG. 9A: Multiple distorted with parenchymal calcification in left kidney with right moderate hydronephrosis.

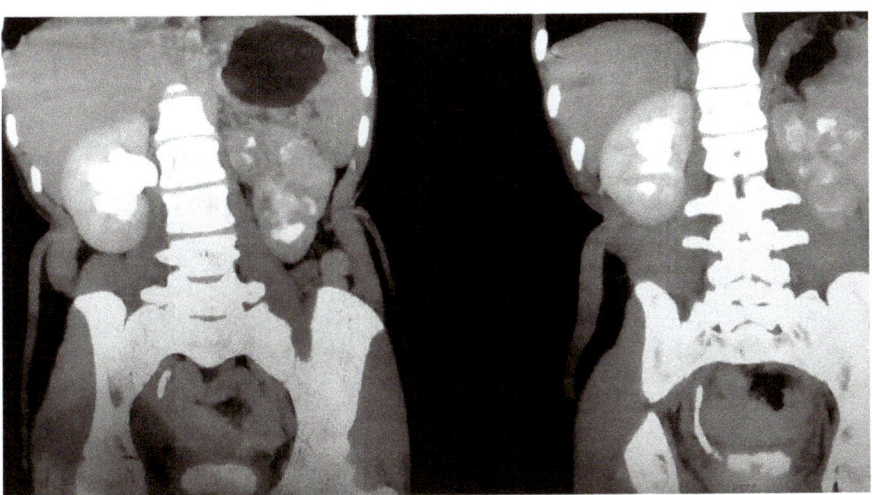

FIG. 9B: Multiple distorted with parenchymal calcification in left kidney with right moderate hydronephrosis.

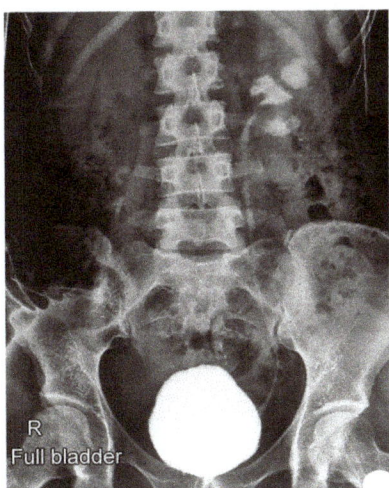

(MCU: micturating cystourethrogram)

FIG. 9C: MCU-full bladder. Left-grade IV reflux with multiple ureteric narrowing with parenchymal calcification with narrow pelvis.

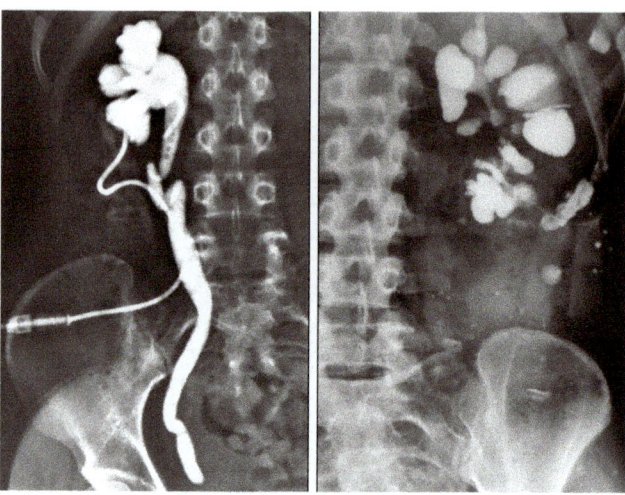

(PCN-O: percutaneous nephrostomy-obstruction)

FIG. 9D: PCN-O gram. Left small pelvis with multiple infundibular stenosis and dilated calyces. Right distal ureteric stricture.

CASE 10

A 28 year-old-female, married, came with history of right flank and lower abdominal pain dull associated with nausea and vomiting. She had repeated febrile UTIs for which she took oral treatment and improved.

No voiding and storage symptoms.

No hematuria.

Four years ago, she was diagnosed to have pulmonary Koch's for which she took AKT for 6 months.

Biochemical investigations normal.

USG: Suggestive of bilateral hydroureteronephrosis with narrowing of middle and distal ureters.

CT urography stricture seen in the upper and lower third segment of the right ureter with proximal mild-to-moderate hydroureteronephrosis and left ureteric narrowing in distal ureter (**Figs. 10A to C**).

Patient underwent bilateral RGP.

Right RGP showed narrowing at midureter with proximal hydronephrosis and for which right DJ stenting was done.

Left RGP showing left lower ureteric narrowing for which DJ stenting was also done. Bladder capacity was 500 cc. Tuberculosis was suspected in view of her past history and repeated UTIs.

Patient was started on Category 1 AKT.

Urinary TB PCR: I/V/O positive (from both the RGP urinary samples).
DTPA renogram (07/09/2015): Left K (GFR)—43.8 mL/min; right K (GFR)—47.8 mL/min.

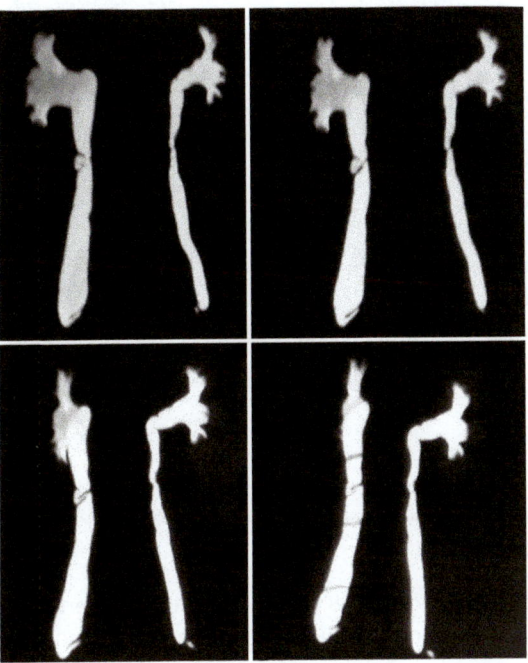

FIG. 10A: Bilateral midureteric strictures with areas of calcification.

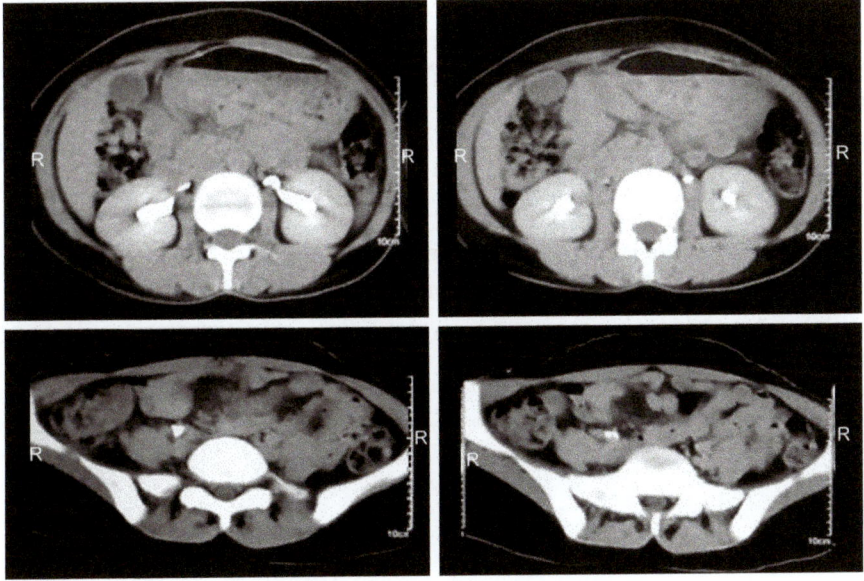

FIG. 10B: Bilateral ureteric calcification and normal pelvicalyceal system.

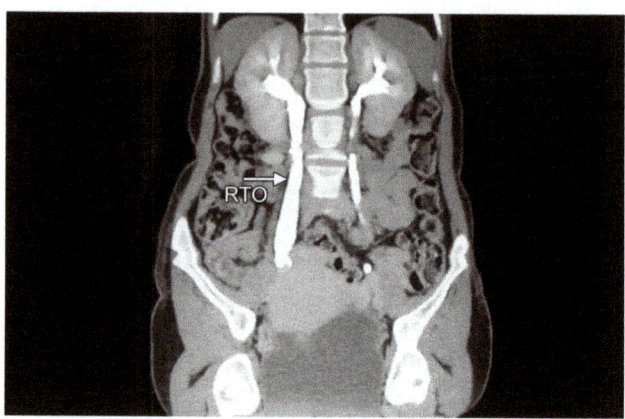

FIG. 10C: Bilateral ureteric strictures in the middle and upper third.

CASE 11

A 36-year-old female, married since 8 years, with primary infertility, presented with left flank pain since 1 year (intermittent, dull aching), frequency and urgency.

No other voiding or storage symptoms.

No h/o uremic symptoms.

History of bilateral tubal block, diagnosed in year 2011 (3 years ago) and taken AKT for 9 months.

Patient's urine culture and sensitivity for MTB complex was positive and patient was started on Category 1 AKT.

Patient underwent left lap nephrectomy on in view of left nonfunctioning kidney (**Fig. 11A**).

H/P report: Tuberculous pyelonephritis.

Material inside kidney sent for culture: Not conclusive of TB.

Cystogram s/o small capacity bladder with right VUR (**Fig. 11B**).

Patient lost follow-up and presented later with h/o AKI, fever, chills for which right PCN insertion was done (**Fig. 11C**). Creatinine was 6.5 mg% which decreased after PCN insertion to 2.7 mg%.

Interesting Cases 139

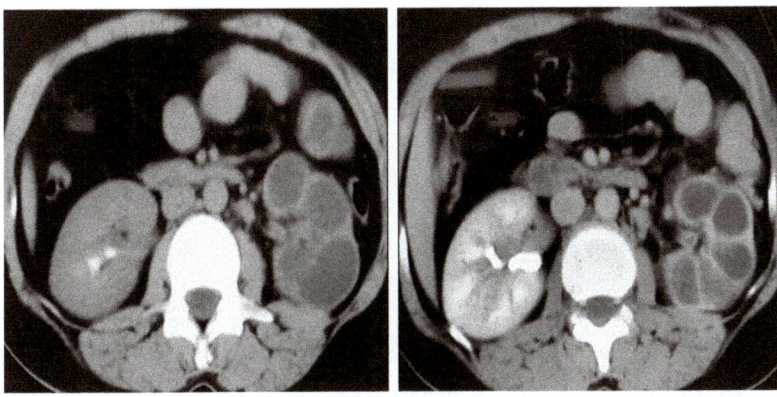

FIG. 11A: Left nonfunctioning kidney with right hydronephrosis (before nephrectomy).

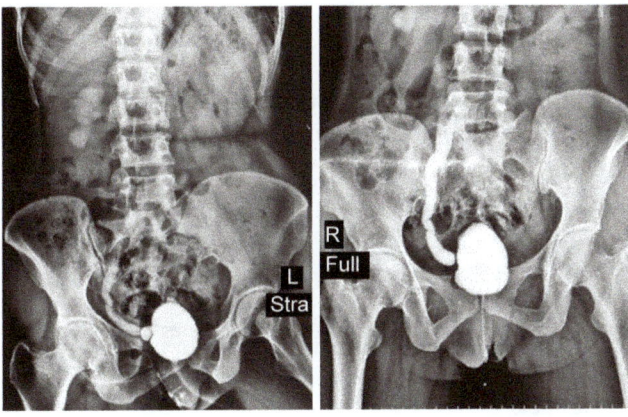

(MCU: micturating cystourethrogram)
FIG. 11B: MCU showing right grade V reflux with vesicoureteric junction stricture with small capacity bladder (after nephrectomy).

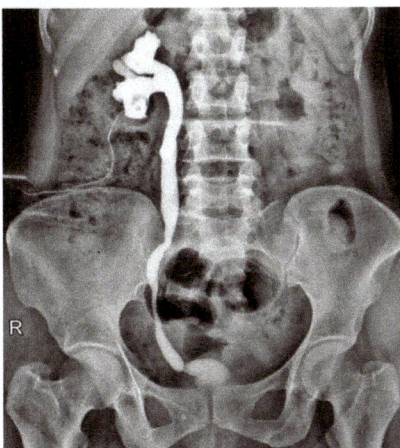

(PCN: percutaneous nephrostomy-obstruction)
FIG. 11C: Right PCN-O-gram showing lower ureteric stricture with small shrunken bladder.

CASE 12

A 12-year-old male patient from Mumbai presented with h/o frequency, urgency, nocturia, and right flank pain since 1 year.

Cough with expectoration and fever since 1.5 months for which patient was investigated and found to have sputum-positive pulmonary Koch's. Patient started on AKT (Category 1).

History of anorexia and weight loss present.

No h/o hematuria/lithuria.

Investigation

Urine R/M: 10–12 RBCs/hpf; 5-6 pus cells/hpf; Bacteria ++.

Urine C/S: Pseudomonas aeruginosa (sensitive to colistin, Imipenem, and polymyxin B).

CBC, LFT, creatinine, and serum electrolytes: Normal.

ESR: 110 mm at end of 1 hour.

Chest X-ray: Large homogenous consolidation present in the right lung field. HRCT chest showed infiltrates present in both lung fields s/o active pulmonary tuberculosis (**Figs. 12 A and B**).

USG: Right moderate HN with HU with thinning of parenchyma; left moderate HN with HU; bladder wall thickened.

GeneXpert detection of TB Sputum: Mycobacterium tuberculosis detected. Rifampicin resistance not detected.

Intravenous pyelography: S/o marked impairment in the function of the right kidney; hydronephrotic changes in the left kidney with fullness of left ureter. Small capacity urinary bladder (**Fig. 12C**).

Urine TB PCR: Positive.

DMSA renogram: Left Kidney shows normal cortical function with dilated PCS. Right kidney is faintly visualized with thin rim of cortex, the function of the kidney is minimal.

Left PCN insertion done.

MCU: S/o thimble bladder with right VUR (**Fig. 12D**).

Left PCN-O-gram: Hold up of contrast at left UV junction suggestive of left lower ureteric stricture. Mildly dilated left PCS (**Fig. 12E**).

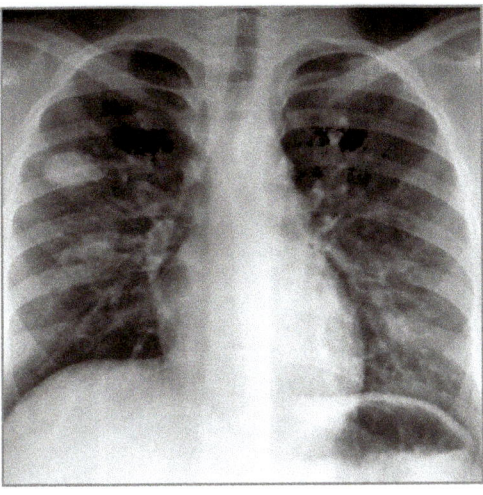

FIG. 12A: Chest X-ray showing large homogenous consolidation in the right lung field. Infiltrates are present in both lung fields suggestive of active pulmonary tuberculosis.

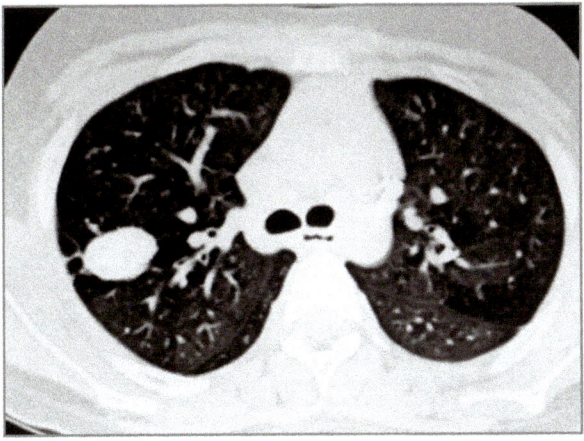

FIG. 12B: HRCT chest showing large homogenous consolidation in the right lung field. Infiltrates are present in both lung fields.

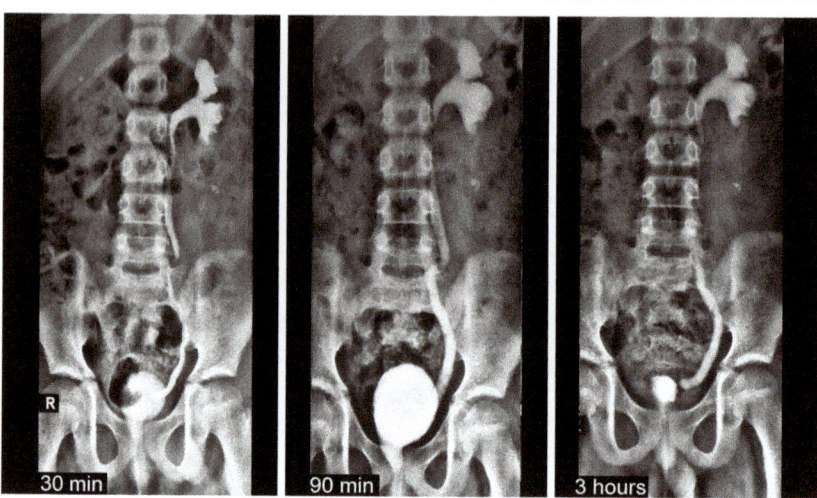

FIG. 12C: Intravenous pyelography: Nonvisualized right kidney with left hydronephrosis and mild ureteric dilatation with left vesicoureteric junction stricture with small capacity urinary bladder.

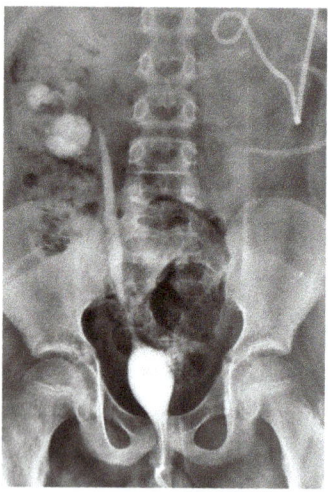

(MCU: micturating cystourethrogram)
FIG. 12D: MCU: Small capacity bladder with right grade 5 reflux.

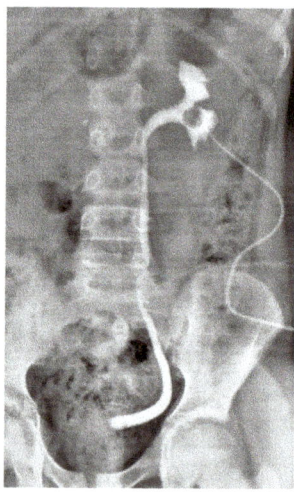

(PCN-O: percutaneous nephrostomy-obstruction)
FIG. 12E: Left PCN-O-gram suggestive of left lower ureteric stricture.

CASE 13

A 24-year-old female, unmarried, presented with h/o frequency, burning micturition, nocturia since 1 month. History of loss of appetite present since 1 year.

Pain in lower abdomen present.

History of fever on and off present.

No h/o lithuria/hematuria.

No prior uro-intervention.

No h/o menstrual irregularities.

Family history: Not contributory.

Investigations

Urine R/M: 8–10 pus cells/hpf.

CBC: 10.3 mg%/7,300.

LFT/RFT/serum electrolytes: Normal.

TB MGIT culture: MPT 64 identification test positive.

Culture positive for Mycobacterium tuberculosis complex.

Sputum AFB: Negative.

Sputum culture: No growth.

Patient started on AKT (Category 1).

USG KUB: Atrophic left kidney. Right kidney-normal; UB: well distended.

CECT: Cross-fused ectopia with lower moiety UPJ obstruction with gross hydronephrosis with abdominal lymphadenopathy (**Fig. 13A**).

EC renogram: Left kidney ectopically positioned attached to lower pole of right kidney. It shows negligible cortical function (<10%). The right kidney shows normal cortical and excretory function.

Intravenous pyelography: Cross fused kidney (**Fig. 13B**) with left kidney fused with right kidney at middle pole with normal functioning right kidney and nonfunctioning fused left moiety.

Urodynamic study: Stable filling phase, poorly compliant bladder, cystometric capacity is 300 mL. Patient voided with good detrusor pressure with good flow rate with PVR-50 mL.

Patient underwent left moiety nephrectomy.

HPR s/o tuberculous pyelonephritis with tuberculous lymphadenitis.

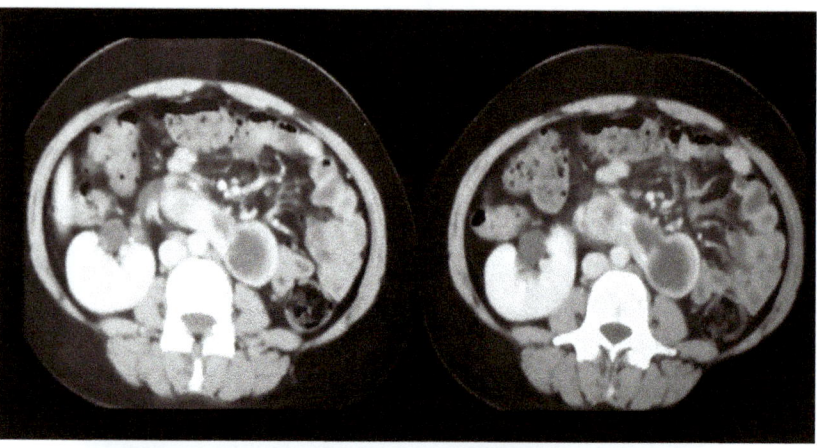

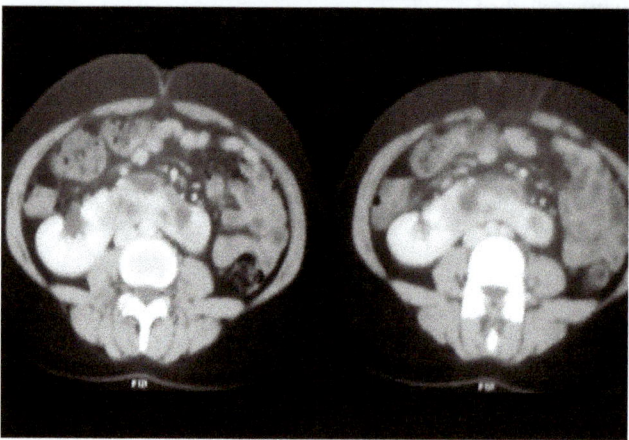

FIG. 13A: Cross-fused ectopia with lower moiety PUJ with gross hydronephrosis with abdominal lymphadenopathy.

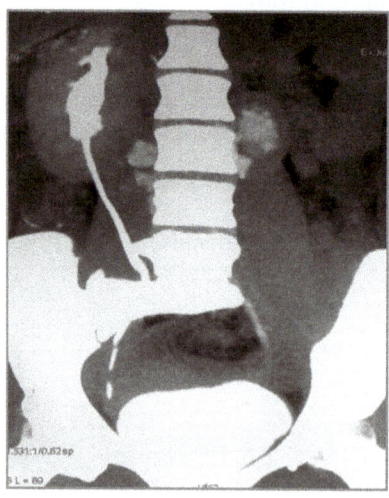

FIG. 13B: Horse shoe kidney with left kidney fused with right kidney at middle pole with normal functioning right kidney and nonfunctioning fused left moiety showing calcification.

CASE 14

A 37-year-old married male patient, presented with h/o frequency of micturition, urgency, dysuria, nocturia since 6 months.

No h/o abdominal pain/nausea/vomiting/fever.

No h/o bowel complaints.

No h/o lithuria/hematuria/pyuria.

Patient started AKT (Category 1) for positive urinary TB PCR done elsewhere.

No h/o pulmonary Koch's/Koch's contact/family history of Koch's.

Bilateral PCN done for raised creatinine.

Investigations

Urine routine/microscopy (13/03/2016): 60–70 pus cells/hpf; 10–15 RBCs/hpf.

ESR: 76 mm at end of 1 hour.

Hb: 9.3; TLC (13/03/2016): 7,600/mm^3.

Urine AFB: Negative.

Urine TB PCR (03/07/2016): Positive.

Serum electrolytes and LFTs: Normal.

Date	16/06/2016	12/07/2016	27/08/2016
Serum creatinine	1.1	1.6	1.2

USG KUB (15/06/2016): Right k-multiple renal cal 4 mm, 7 mm, 5 mm, and 6 mm.

Left mid ureteric obstructing cal 7 mm with proximal hydroureteronephrosis.

*X KUB (***Fig. 14 A***)* showed right renal parenchymal calcifications with multiple right renal calculi and left upper ureteric calculi at L4 level.

CT IVU (20/07/2016): Right multiple renal calculus with hydronephrosis (**Fig. 14B**); Left upper ureteric 8 mm cal with proximal hydroureteronephrosis. There is distortion of renal parenchymal architecture along with pelvicalyceal system. There is also periureteric fat stranding with thickened ureteric walls (**Fig. 14C**). Bladder appears small contracted and thick walled with altered contour suggestive of tuberculous cystitis (**Fig. 14D**).

Patient is lost to follow-up.

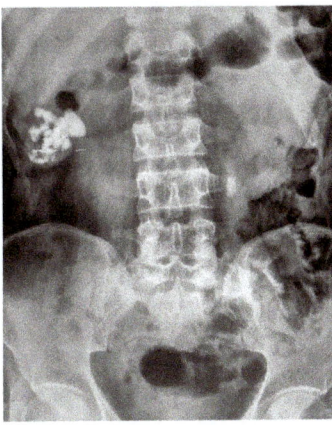

FIG.14A: X-ray KUB suggestive of right renal calculus with parenchymal calcification and left ureteric calculus.

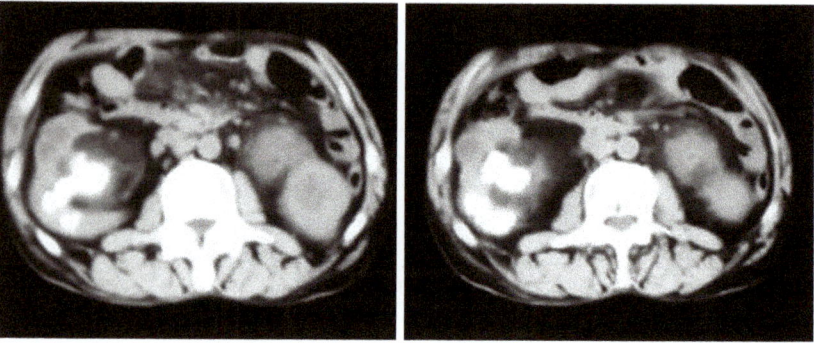

FIG. 14B: Right multiple renal calculus with hydronephrosis with left upper ureteric 8 mm calculus with proximal hydroureteronephrosis.

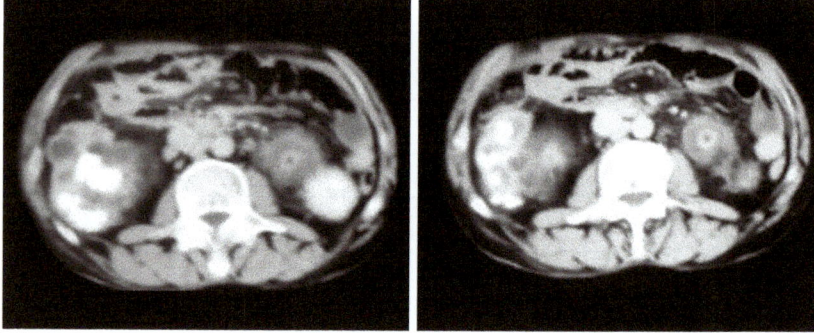

FIG. 14C: Right distorted pelvicalyceal system with parenchymal calcification with dilated ureters.

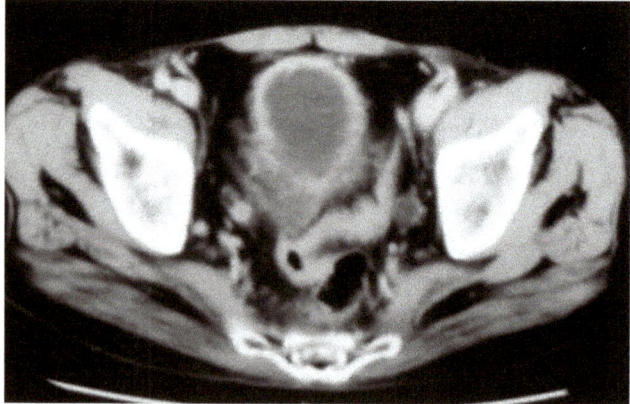

FIG. 14D: Thick walled bladder with dilated thick walled distal ureter.

CASE 15

A 38-year-old female married since 20 years having 3 issues, r/o Wadala, Mumbai presented with right flank pain dull intermittent along with h/o dysuria/frequency/nocturia since 3 months. Patient evaluated for the same and found to have right lower ureteric calculus with left renal calculus. She underwent right URSL but intraoperatively found to have multiple tubercles in the bladder. Hence, biopsy of tubercles was taken along with bilateral ureteral urine samples. Patient started on Category 1 as biopsy s/o tuberculosis. Urine showed pyuria with sterile culture. Her CBC, RFT, LFT, and serum electrolytes were normal. Her urine AFB smear (from bilateral ureteral samples) and urine TB PCR were negative.

On USG KUB: Right k-moderate hydronephrosis with hydroureter up to iliac crest. Left K-8 mm upper pole calculus seen with focal calyectasis; UB: well distended.

On CT IVU: 5 mm calculus is seen in right ureter at pelvic brim with proximal hydroureteronephrosis (**Figs. 15A and B**). 10 mm calculus is seen in mid-pole and 7 mm at lower pole of left kidney. Both kidneys are normal in functioning (**Figs. 15C and D**).

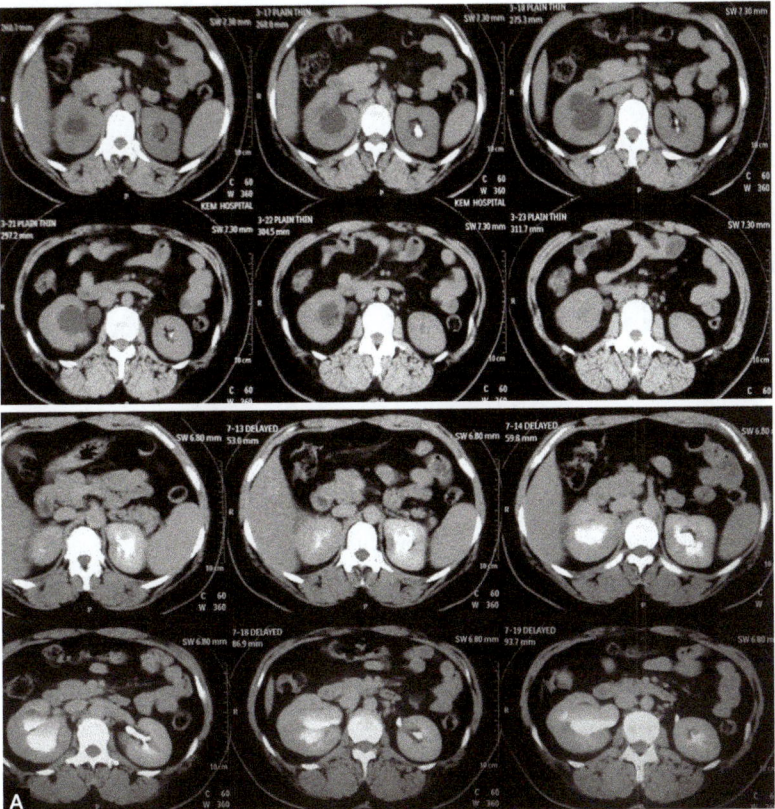

FIGS. 15A AND B:

Continued...

Continued...

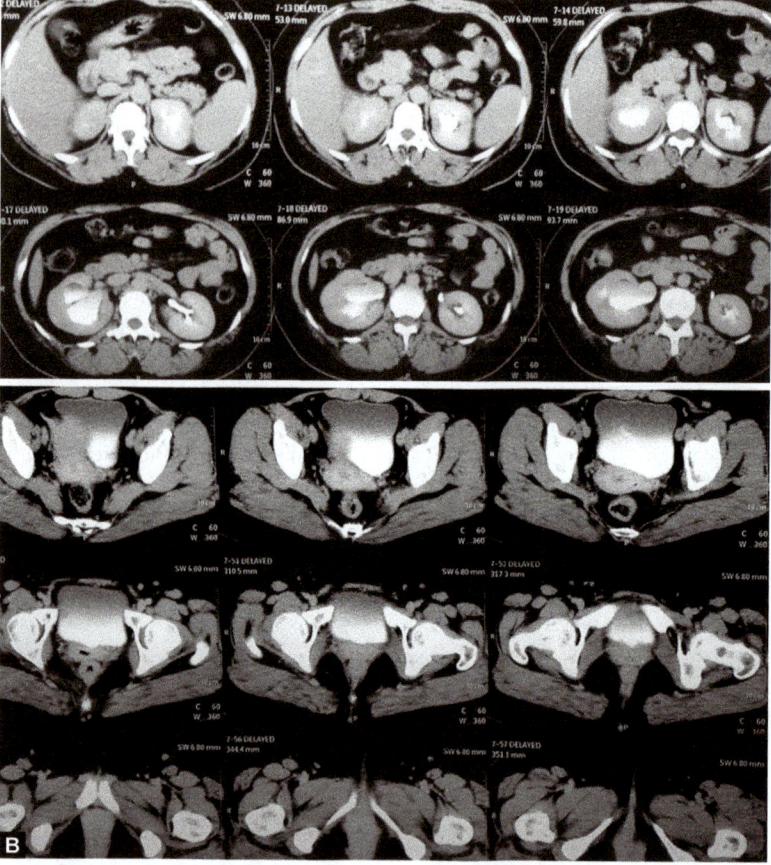

FIGS. 15A AND B: About 5 mm calculus is seen in right ureter at pelvic brim with proximal hydroureteronephrosis. About 10 mm calculus is seen in mid-pole and 7 mm at lower pole of left kidney.

*Intravenous pyelography (**Figs. 15E, F, and G**):* Normal functioning both kidneys with right kidney showing irregular hydronephrosis with narrow infundibulum. Left kidney shows moderate hydronephrosis with narrow infundibulum.

*MCU (**Figs. 15H and I**):* Normal capacity bladder with smooth outline. No e/o reflux seen. No post-void residue present.

Patient started on Category 1 AKT and underwent right miniperc for the renal calculi. Post PCNL she is lost to follow-up.

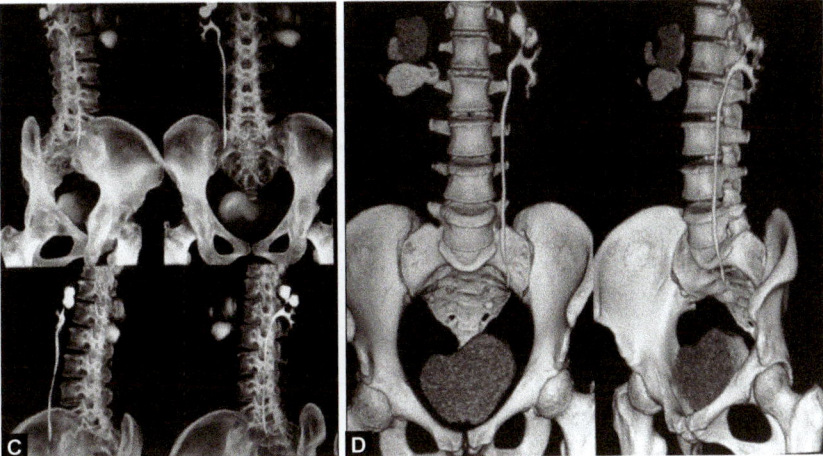

FIGS. 15C AND D: Urography images showing normal excretion from both kidneys with right moderate HN with distorted PCS and left superior calyceal infundibular stenosis.

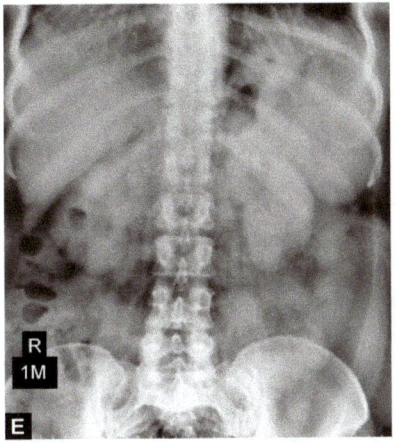

FIG. 15E: Image showing nephrogram phase of IVP.

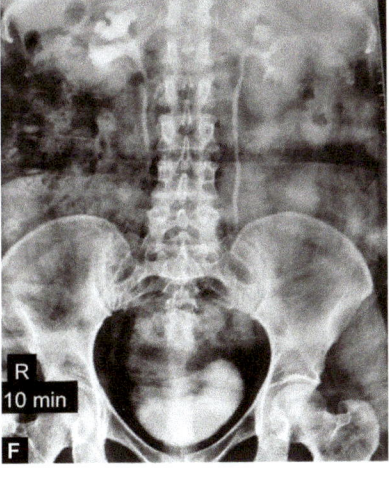

FIG. 15F: Image showing excretory phase of IVP with right moderate HN with infundibular stenosis with left superior hydrocalycosis.

Continued

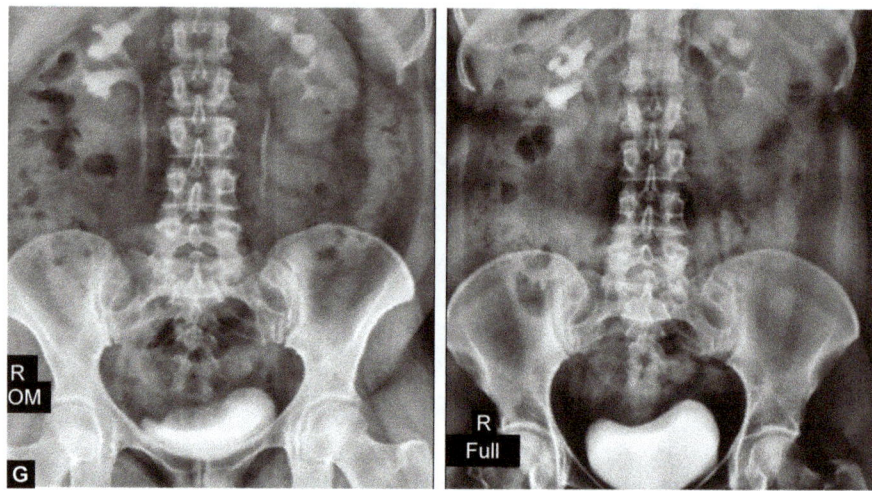

FIGS. 15G: Intravenous pyelography (29/08/16).

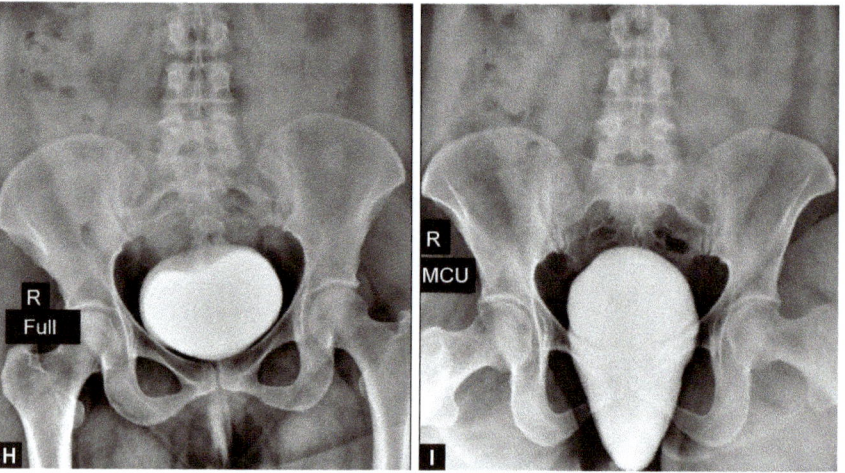

FIGS. 15H AND I: MCU (28/08/2016).

CASE 16

A 25-year-old female, married since 6 years presented with.

Left flank pain dull aching continuous since 3–4 years.

No h/o dysuria/frequency/nocturia.

No h/o fever/weight loss/loss of appetite.

Patient was evaluated and found to have left side hydronephrosis with PUJ calculus of size 1 cm (**Fig. 16A**).

Urine pregnancy test was positive (March, 2015).

Patient was advised left DJ stenting i/v/o raised serum creatinine (1.42 mg%) and persistent left flank but patient was unwilling for the same.

Normal delivery took place with healthy male child.

Patient was followed up immediately after delivery with further raised serum creatinine 1.8 mg% and CT findings s/o left side hydronephrosis with calcification and calculus and right side hydrocalycosis (**Fig. 16B**). Patient underwent cystourethroscopy with bilateral RGP. Bladder mucosa was edematous inflamed and right RGP showing hydrocalycosis with infundibular stenosis and upper ureteric narrowing. Left RGP s/o infundibular stenosis with hydrocalycosis with calcification. Bilateral DJ stenting done along with bilateral ureteral urine samples sent for TB smear and culture.

Patient started on Category 1 on January, 2016 but was lost follow-up in between.

Patient underwent medical termination of second pregnancy in May, 2016.

Patient has completed AKT on June, 2016.

Family history: Not contributory.

Obstetric history: P2L1A1.

No h/o menstrual irregularities.

No past h/o pulmonary Koch's or Koch's contact.

O/E-Vitals: Stable.

No pallor.

Systemic examination: NAD.

Investigations

Urine R/M (10/08/2015): 15-20 pus cells/hpf.

Urine C/S- (26/10/2015): No growth.

Urine R/M (16/08/2016): 3–4 pus cells/hpf; 1–2 RBCs/hpf.

Urine C/S (24/08/2016): No growth.

Hb: 10.2 g%; TLC: 7,900/mm^3.

Date	19/03/15	9/05/15	16/11/15	01/03/16	12/08/16
Serum creatinine	1.42	1.6	1.8 Bilateral DJ stenting done	1.38	1.7
BUN	25	28.0	34.4	24.3	27

LFT and serum electrolytes: Normal.

CT KUB (Plain): Bilateral hydronephrosis with thinning of renal parenchyma with multiple parenchymal calcification and cortical abscess seen.

UB: Distended; Normal.

Urine AFB: Positive.

Urine AFB culture: No growth.

Patient underwent bilateral PCN as repeat RGP showed significant stricture involving bilateral middle and lower third ureters.

Patient underwent rat tail anastomosis for bilateral long segment ureteric strictures.

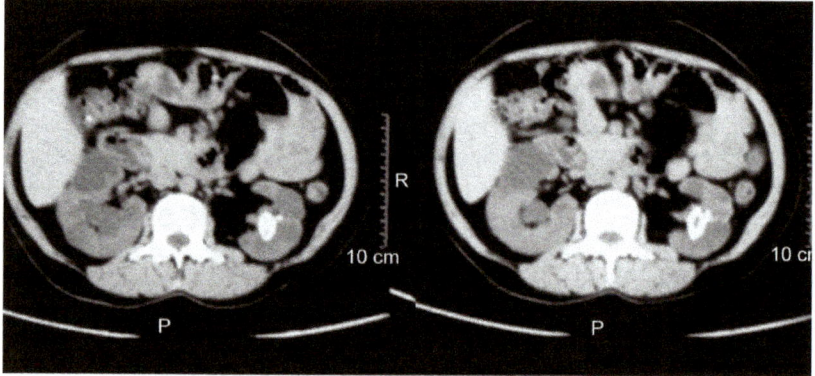

FIG. 16A: Hypodense areas in upper and middle pole of right kidney with parenchymal calcification with left PUJ calculus with hypodense areas.

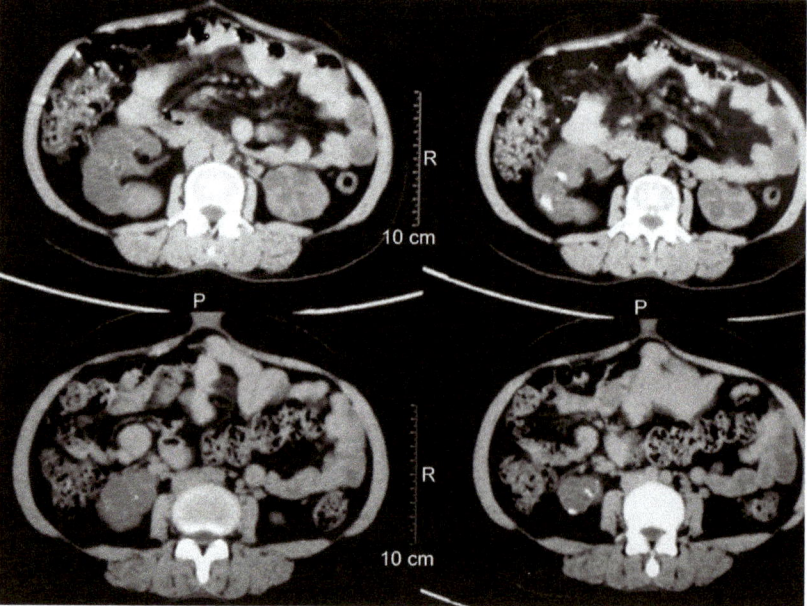

FIG. 16B: Hydronephrotic right kidney with distorted parenchymal architecture and PC system with calcifications in the parenchyma.

CASE 17

A 18-year-old unmarried male, r/o Bandra presented with history of swelling on the undersurface of the penis and right inguinal region for 1 year.

No h/o pain/trauma/fever.

No h/o frequency/urgency/dysuria.

No h/o weight loss/loss of appetite.

No past h/o pulmonary Koch's or Koch's contact.

O/E-Vitals: Stable.

No pallor.

Local Examination: 2 × 2 cm size firm, non-tender nodular lesion present on the undersurface of penis, overlying skin is normal (**Figs. 17A and B**). Left epididymal head is nodular and non-tender. Right inguinal lymph nodes multiple, firm, and non-tender of size approx. 2 × 1.5 cm is largest.

Investigations

Urine R/M (22/12/2015): 1–2 pus cells/hpf.

Urine C/S: No growth.

Hb:13.2 g%; TLC: 7,900/mm^3.

RFTs, LFTs, and serum electrolytes: Normal.

Urine AFB: No AFB seen.

Urine AFB culture: No growth.

FNAC of penile lesion (08/12/2015): Abundant necrosis and calcified material with occasional histiocytes.

FNAC of right inguinal lymph node (08/12/2015): Necrotizing granulomatous lymphadenitis.

USG KUB: Both kidneys normal in size and shape.

UB: Well distended.

*Intravenous pyelography (**Fig. 17C**)*: Both kidneys normal in size and shape. No e/o hydroureteronephrosis. UB appears normal.

RGU: Normal.

Swelling subsided but not resolved with CAT 1 AKT for 9 months.

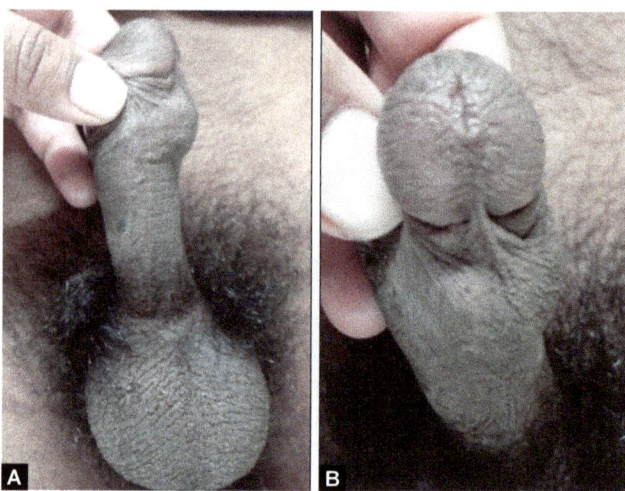

FIGS. 17A AND B: Picture showing nodular lesion present on the ventral surface of penis.

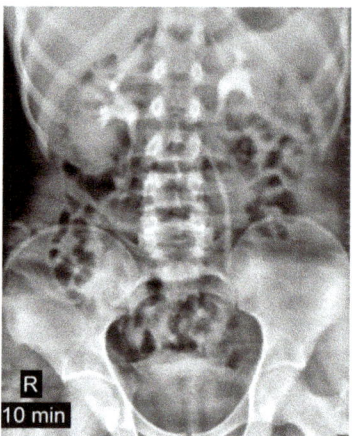

FIG. 17C: Normal intravenous pyelography.

CASE 18

A 60-year-old female, married resident of Uttar Pradesh presented with c/o.

Continuous urinary incontinence for 1 year with daily 5 pads changes, urgency and frequency and dysuria for 2 years.

History of weight loss since 2 years associated with anorexia.

Patient was evaluated and found to have bilateral hydroureteronephrosis with small capacity bladder with fistulous communication between bladder and vagina and Urine TB PCR was positive. Patient started on Category 1 AKT.

History of tubal ligation 10 years back.

Open cholecystectomy 25 years back.

k/c/o epileptic disorder since 7–8 years.

No h/o TB or TB contact.

Not k/c/o DM/HTN or any other medical illness.

No h/o radiation.

No h/o abdominal/genital region trauma.

No h/o any menstrual cycle complaints.

Normal obstetric history with 6 live issues.

All full-term normal vaginal delivery.

No ANC or PNC complications.

Menopause for 15 years.

O/E-Vitals: Stable.

No pallor.

Local examination: Defect present along anterior vaginal wall with continuous dribbling of urine. On cystoscopy approximately 2.5 × 2.0 cm defect present in supratrigonal region with small capacity bladder of approximately 50 cc.

Systemic examination: NAD.

Investigations

Urine R/M: 8–10 pus cells/hpf.

Urine C/S: No growth.

Hb: 11.0 g%; TLC: 5,600/mm^3; Lymphocytes: 30%.

Serum creatinine: 1.0 mg%; BUN: 9.0.

LFT and serum electrolytes: Normal.

Urine AFB: Negative.

Urine AFB culture: No growth.

Urine TB PCR-Positive (All three samples).

Micturating cystourethrogram: Small capacity bladder with right grade 3 reflux and left grade 2 reflux (**Fig. 18A**). Fistulous communication between urinary bladder and vagina. Distorted tortuous right lower ureter with multiple ill-defined blind ending sinus tracts

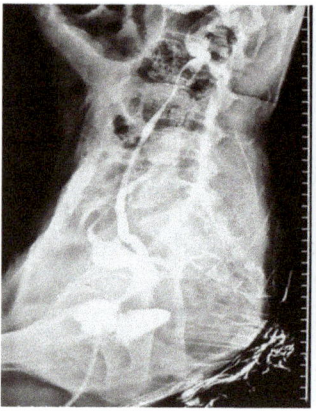
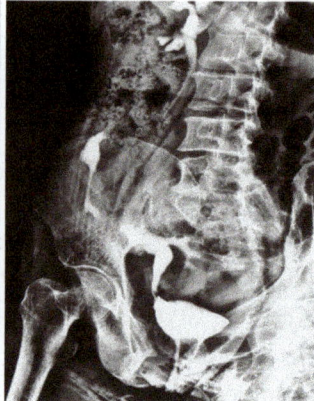

FIG.18A: MCU-Small capacity bladder with right grade 3 reflux and left grade 2 reflux. Fistulous communication between urinary bladder and vagina. Distorted tortuous right lower ureter with multiple ill-defined blind ending sinus tracts arising from it and radiating in different directions.

arising from it and radiating in different directions-likely to be sequel of postoperative ureteric injury.

Intravenous pyelography: Bilateral normal functioning kidneys. Moderate–gross dilatation of left pelvicalyceal system and the ureter in entire extent up to UB (**Fig. 18B**). Well demarcated defect in the mid portion of right renal pelvis with effacement of adjacent calyces, due to mid pole renal lesion. Distorted tortuous right lower ureter with multiple ill-defined blind ending sinus tracts arising from it and radiating in different directions-likely to be sequel of postoperative ureteric injury.

CECT (abdomen and pelvis): Bilateral hydroureteronephrosis. Renal parenchyma is well opacified. About 3 mm defect noted between floor of urinary bladder and anterior wall of vagina. Sinus tract along right lateral wall of pelvis communicating with right lower ureter, no communication with bowel (**Figs. 18C to E**).

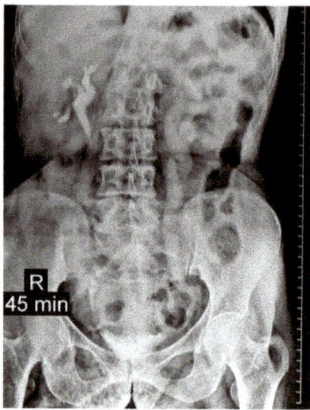
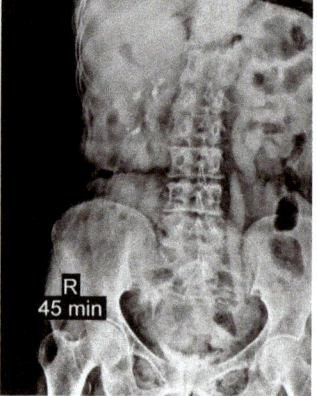

FIG. 18B: Normal right pelvicalyceal system with dilated left pelvicalyceal system and ureter. Right lower ureter narrow, not properly delineated.

Interesting Cases

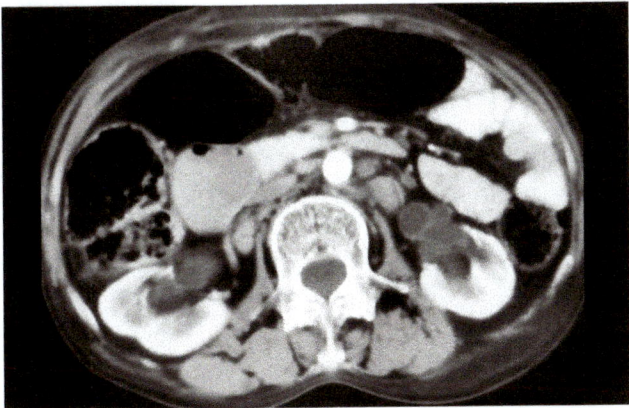

FIG. 18C: Left hydronephrosis.

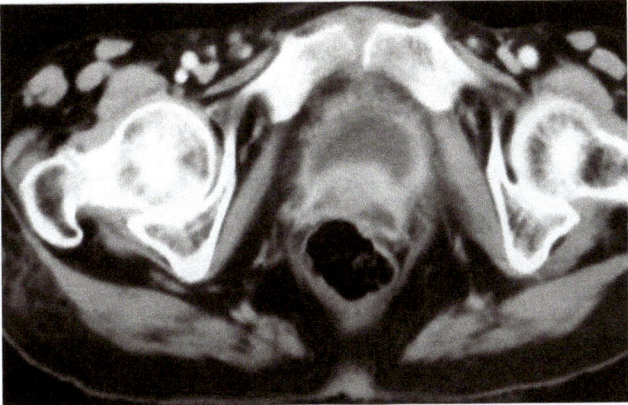

FIG. 18D: Thickened bladder and contrast in vagina.

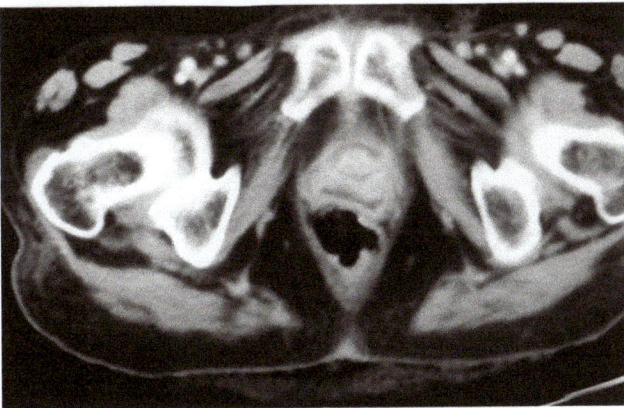

FIG. 18E: Small contracted bladder and contrast in vagina.

Exploratory laparotomy showed entire distal small intestine studded with tubercles (**Fig. 18F**). Uterovesical fold dissected to open the bladder. Inside the bladder was unhealthy mucosa with defect of 2.5 × 2.5 cm with contracted small-sized bladder (**Fig. 18G**). Cystectomy with hysterectomy was done as the bladder was friable and could not hold sutures. Vaginal cuff was closed with difficulty. Ileal conduit surgery was performed using the proximal ileum.

H/P report: Necrotizing tissue with granulomatous reaction suggestive of tuberculosis.

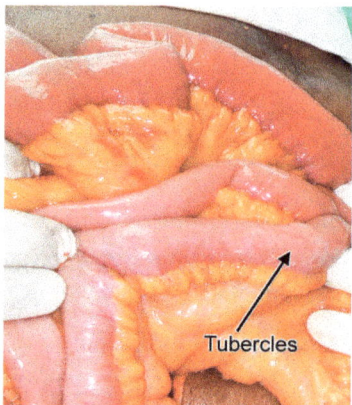

FIG. 18F: Picture showing ileum studded with tubercles.

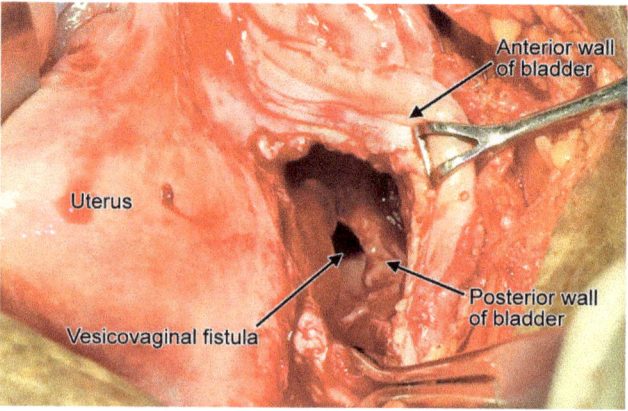

FIG. 18G: Picture showing large vesicovaginal fistula (VVF) with unhealthy bladder.

CASE 19

A 40-year-old male, married for 16 years, having three issues, Hindu, r/o Mumbai, presented with c/o.

Increased daytime frequency of urination, dysuria, and nocturia since 6 months.

History of straining, intermittency during micturition relieved on alpha-blockers since 6 months.

No h/o fever/weight loss/loss of appetite/flank pain.

No h/o prior pulmonary Koch's/Koch's contact.

No h/o decreased ejaculation.

O/E-vitals: Stable.

DRE: Firm grade III prostate with irregular surface; mucosa free.

Testis/Epididymis/Vas: Normal.

Investigations

Urine R/M: 15–20 Pus cells/hpf.

Urine C/S: No growth.

Urine AFB: AFB not seen.

Urine TB PCR: Negative.

Serum PSA: 6.31 ng/mL.

Hb: 12.7 g%; *TLC*: 9,900/mm^3; *ESR*: 12 mm at the end of 1 hour.

Serum electrolytes, LFTs, and RFTs-WNL.

HIV/HBsAg/Anti-HCV: Negative.

USG KUB: Both kidneys normal in size, shape. No e/o hydro-ureteronephrosis. *UB*: Partially distended; wall thickened. Prostate moderately enlarged, heterogeneous echotexture with ill-defined margins, approximately of size 4.9 × 5.2 × 4.7 cm.

Patient underwent TRUS guided biopsy of prostate (**Fig. 19A**). H/P Report ill-defined epitheloid cell granulomas suggestive of tuberculosis.

MCU showing well distended bladder with smooth outlines. Capacity appears adequate without any reflux, mass or diverticuli (**Fig. 19B**).

AKT Category 1 advised for 9 months. Patient lost to follow-up.

Genitourinary Tuberculosis

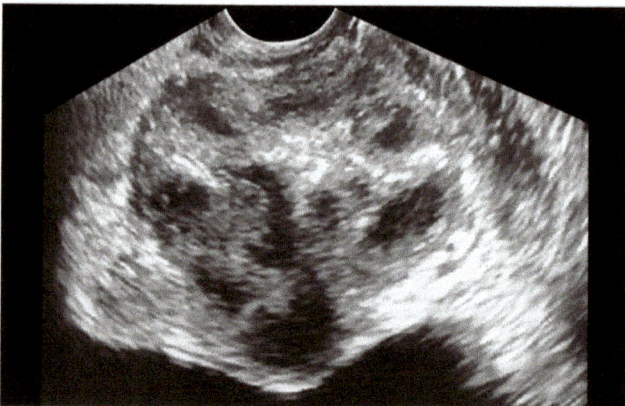

FIG. 19A: TRUS-Prostate gland measures 6.1 × 5.3 × 4.7 cm corresponding to 82 g. Multiple hypoechoic masses with cystic changes noted s/o abscesses measuring 1 or 2 cm occupying entire gland.

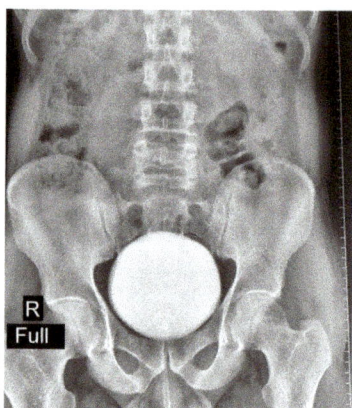

FIG. 19B: MCU-Bladder is well distended with smooth wall. Urethra normal. No e/o reflux seen.

CASE 20

A 22-year-old female married for 3 years, r/o Andheri presented with.

Increased frequency of micturition, urgency, dysuria, and pyuria since 8–9 months.

C/o suprapubic pain dull aching, intermittent which increases during micturition since 8–9 months.

No h/o fever/weight loss/loss of appetite.

No h/o prior uro-intervention.

Patient was evaluated and found to have focal upper pole cortical thinning in the left kidney with superior pole hydrocalycosis. Patient was started on Category 1 in view of positive urine TB PCR.

Obstetric history: History of two abortions.

Patient underwent left DJ stenting under anesthesia for left hydronephrosis and left flank pain. Her symptoms relieved after the same. Left DJ stent removed after 6 weeks and symptoms recurred.

No comorbidity.

O/E-Vitals: Stable.

S/E-NAD.

Investigations

Urine R/M: 20–25 pus cells/hpf.

Urine C/S: No growth.

CBC: Hb: 13.2 g%; TLC: 4,600/mm^3.

ESR: 64 mm at the end of 1 hour.

RFTs, LFTs, and serum electrolytes: Normal.

Urine AFB: Not seen.

Urine AFB Culture: No growth seen.

Urine TB PCR: Positive (two samples).

Drug sensitivity: Not done.

USG KUB: Right K: Normal; Left K: Focal upper pole cortical thinning with superior pole hydrocalycosis; UB: Normal.

CT IVU (**Figs. 20A and B**): Right K: Normal functioning and normal size. Left K: Infundibular stenosis in superior calyx with hydrocalycosis of the upper pole.

Patient underwent left upper pole nephrectomy i/v/o persistent left flank pain.

H/P report of specimen: Interstitial tissue showing dense lymphocytic infiltration but no e/o granuloma or caseation seen. F/s/o chronic pyelonephritis.

At present patient is asymptomatic.

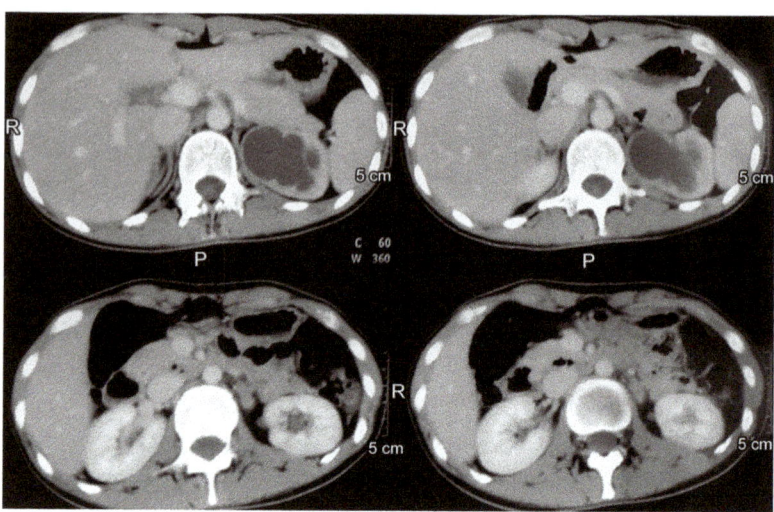

FIG. 20A: CT IVU: Dilatation of the left upper calyx selectively.

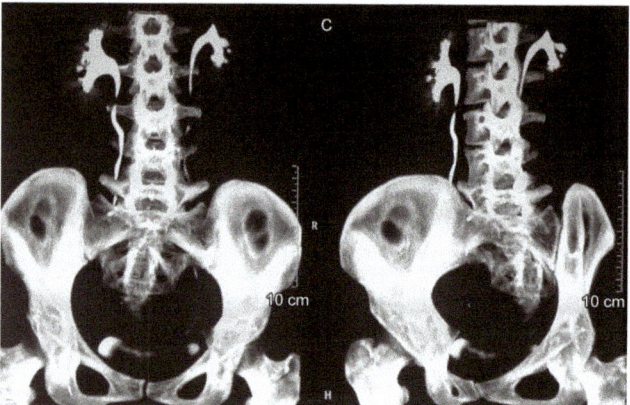

FIG. 20B: Left upper phantom calyx.

CASE 21

A 45-year-old female, married having six issues, r/o Madhya-Pradesh presented with c/o.
Increased frequency of urination, dysuria, and nocturia for 1 year.
History of occasional right flank pain mild in intensity present.
No h/o fever/weight loss/loss of appetite.
History of right open pyelolithotomy 2 years back.
History of left PCNL 1 year back.
Patient was evaluated for the same. Imaging s/o right k-gross hydronephrosis with intrarenal pelvis with complete cut-off at upper ureter L1 level. Cystoscopy s/o small capacity bladder with bilateral golf-hole ureteric orifices. Patient underwent bilateral RGP with left DJ stenting and right PCN. Patient was started on Category 1 on 13/05/2016 i/v/o Imaging and cystoscopy findings.
k/c/o DM on regular insulin.
O/E-Vitals: Stable.
S/E-NAD.

Investigations

Urine R/M: 20–25 pus cells/hpf; 4–5 RBCs/hpf.
Urine C/S: No growth.
Hb: 8.3 g%; *TLC*: 8,900/mm^3.
ESR-71 mm at the end of 1 hour.

Date	05/04/16	06/04/16	18/04/16	25/04/16	15/05/16
Serum creatinine	6.32	4.42	4.8	5.4	4.1

USG KUB (04/04/2016): Right K-Gross hydronephrosis with paper thin parenchyma; Left K: Increased echotexture with multiple simple cortical cysts. UB: Minimally distended.

Patient underwent cystoscopy with bilateral RGP on 05/04/2016. Findings s/o small capacity bladder with bilateral golf-hole ureteric orifices with complete cut-off at L1 level right upper ureter. Left mild hydronephrosis with entire hydroureter. Contrast not draining into the bladder. Patient underwent left DJ stenting and right PCN.

Right PCN-O-gram (19/04/2016) (**Figs. 21A and B**): Gross hydronephrosis with intrarenal pelvis. Right ureter not opacified.
Right PCN o/p: 500 mL/24 h.
Per urethral o/p: 1,500 mL/24 h.
Urine AFB (29/04/2016): Negative.
Urine AFB culture (14/06/2016): No growth.
Urine TB PCR (25/04/2016): Negative.
MCU (09/05/2016) (**Figs. 21C and D**): Small capacity UB with irregular bladder walls (**Fig. 21E**). Right V-U reflux with moderately dilated tortuous right ureter with abrupt cut-off at PUJ. Left grade III reflux with blunting of calyces.

Patient underwent right nephron ureterectomy after 4 weeks of AKT.

HPR suggestive of granulomatous infiltration: TB.

Serum creatinine continues to be high and further management in view of future renal replacement therapy refused by patient.

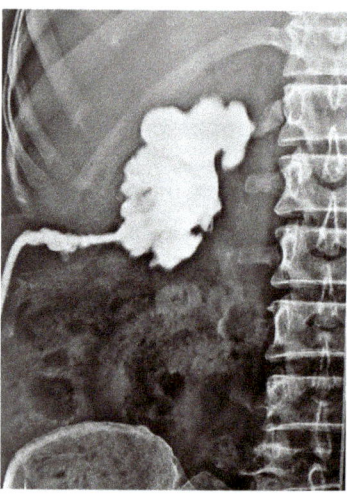

FIG. 21A: Right PCN-O-gram showing intrarenal pelvis with narrowing at the PUJ with no contrast entering the ureter.

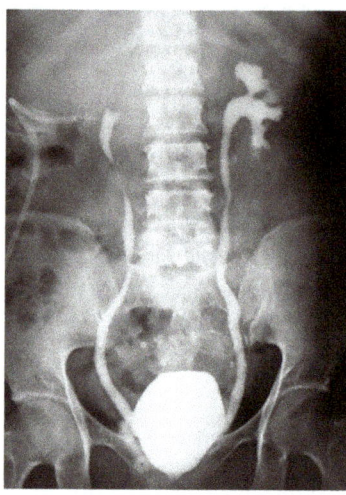

FIG. 21B: MCU-bilateral reflux with small capacity bladder with right PCN with no contrast entering the right renal pelvis.

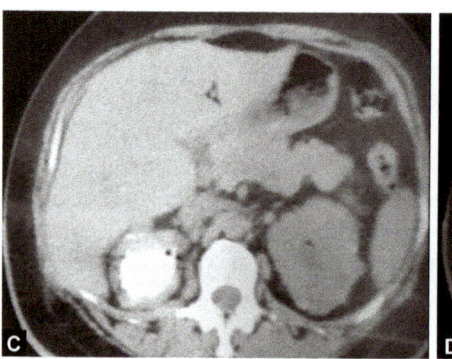

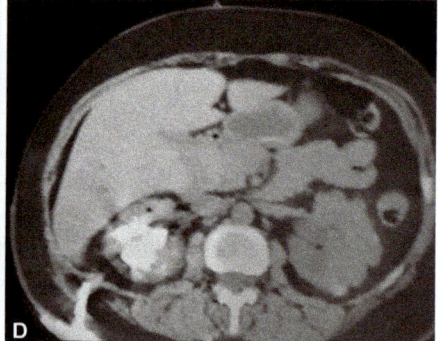

FIGS. 21C AND D: CT PCN gram showing dilated right pelvicalyceal system with parenchymal calcification.

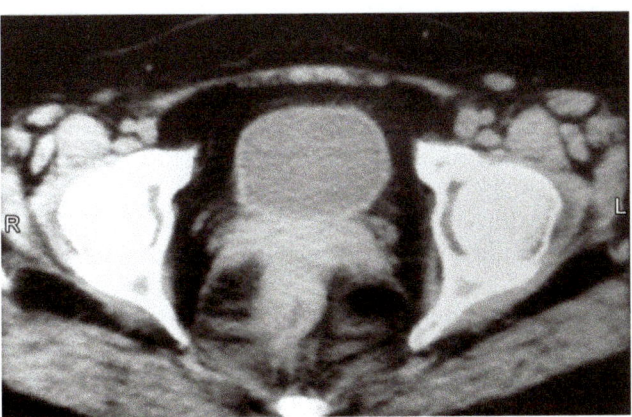
FIG. 21E: Thickened bladder.

CASE 22

Clinical Presentation
Afzal, 28-year male, resident of Gonda, UP presented with history of passing urine per rectally and painless bothersome leakage of urine through opening in perineum accompanied by urgency for 3 years.

Treatment History
Patient underwent colonoscopy for above complaints and was diagnosed with prostatorectal fistula. Patient underwent transperineal prostrate rectal fistula repair with sigmoid colostomy and SPC in December, 2015. Followed by postoperative wound dehiscence and perineal urine leakage 2 weeks post procedure. Patient underwent colonoscopy in October, 2016 and was detected with recurrence of fistula.

Examination
Scarred perineum with two openings in perineum at 5 and 7 o'clock positions.

Laboratory Investigations

Serum creatinine: 1.1 mg/dL.
Urine analysis: 3–4 pus cells, no growth.
Patient was started on CAT 1 AKT for 6 months after which the fistulae healed, however, AKT was continued for 6 months more before surgery.

Cystoscopy December, 2017
- Anterior urethra healthy.
- Per urethral scope could not be negotiated beyond prostatic urethra impression of veru seen.
- *SPC scopy:* Bladder neck open and neck multiple fibrous tracts beyond the bladder.
- Biopsy taken and sent for HPE.
- Guidewire negotiated across bladder neck came out through perineum at 5 o' clock position.
- Methylene blue inserted through SPC, presence of methylene blue in anal canal 2 cm from anal orifice.
- e/o two vesical calculi 1 cm in size PCCL done.

Cystoscopy April, 2018
- Penile urethra normal.
- Scope could not be negotiated beyond midbulbar urethra GW could not be passed beyond.
- 17 Fr 30° SPC scopy done.
- Bladder neck open. Multiple septae and flakes seen distal to veru guidewire comes out of the anal opening and not the perineum.
- Water leaking through anal opening around the guidewire.

Treatment

Patient underwent prostatectomy and urethral fistula excision and vesicourethral anastomosis (**Figs. 22A to G**).

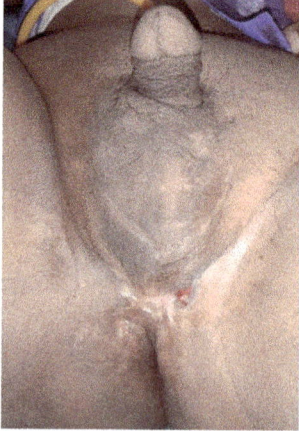

FIG. 22A: Perineal picture showing empty scrotum with scars and multiple fistula.

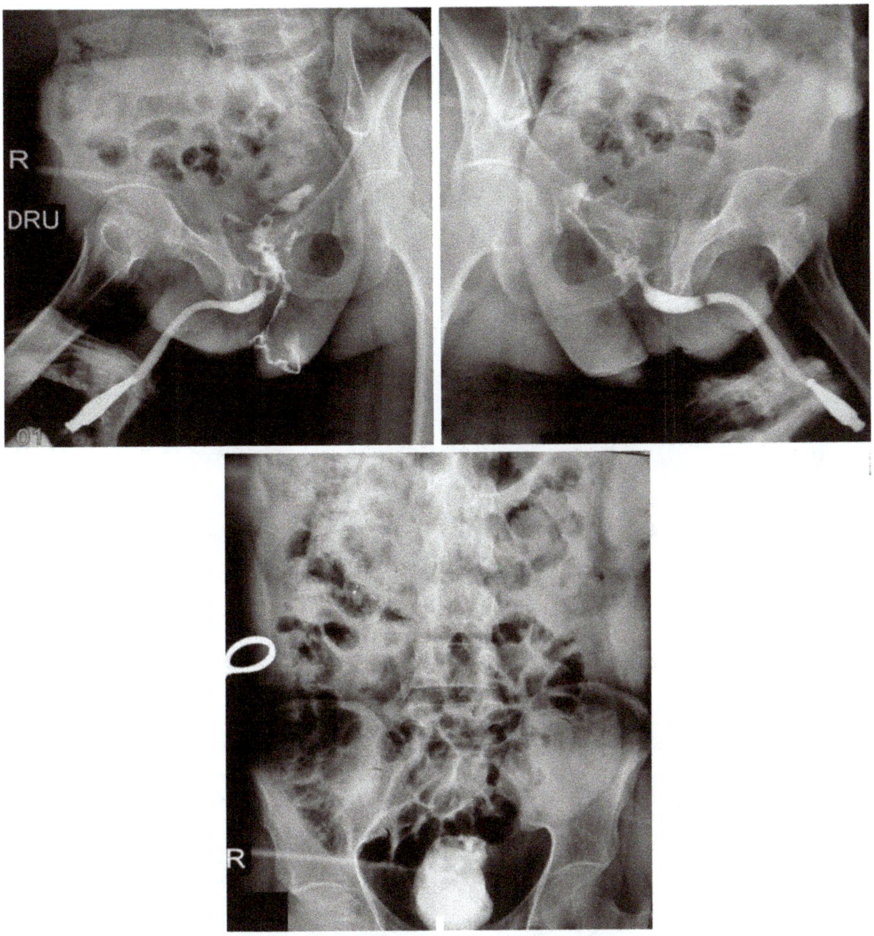

FIG. 22B: MCU/RGU prostatic–rectal fistula with cutaneous fistula.

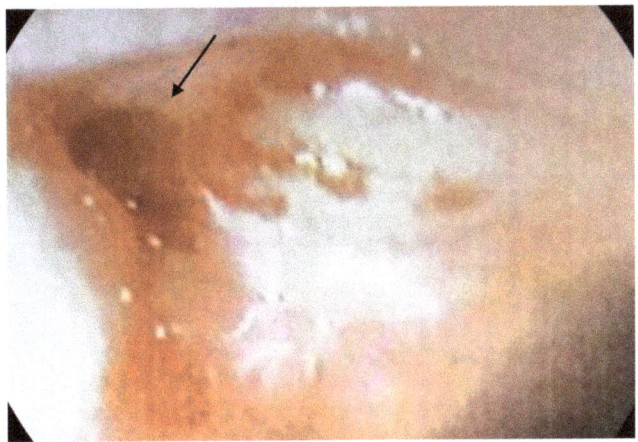

FIG. 22C: Colonoscopy showing rectal opening of the fistula.

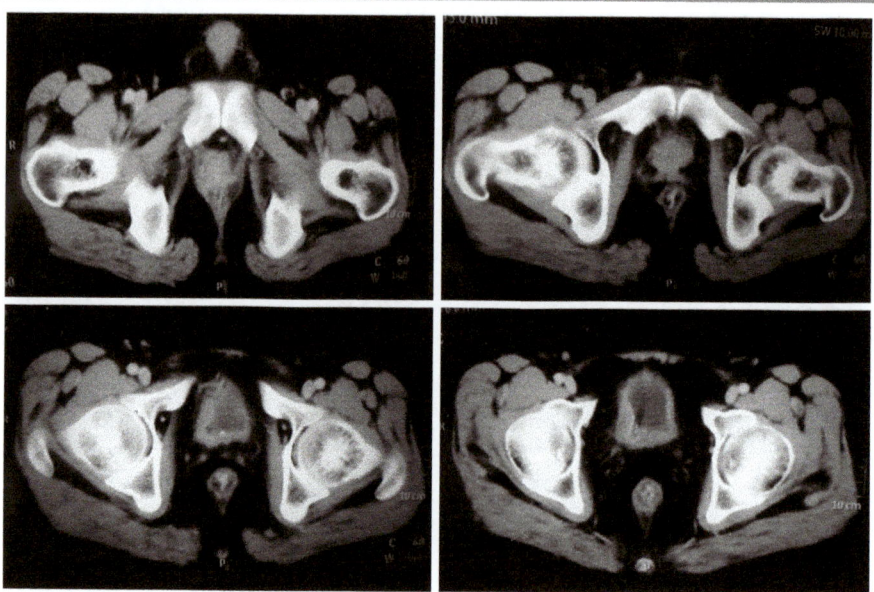

FIG. 22D: CT IVU post AKT showing destroyed prostatic architecture with hypodense areas, calcification, and air.

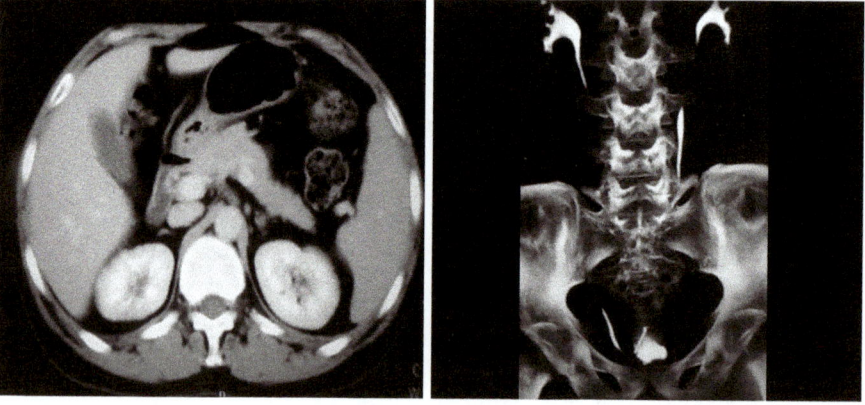

FIG. 22E: Normal pelvicalyceal system on both sides.

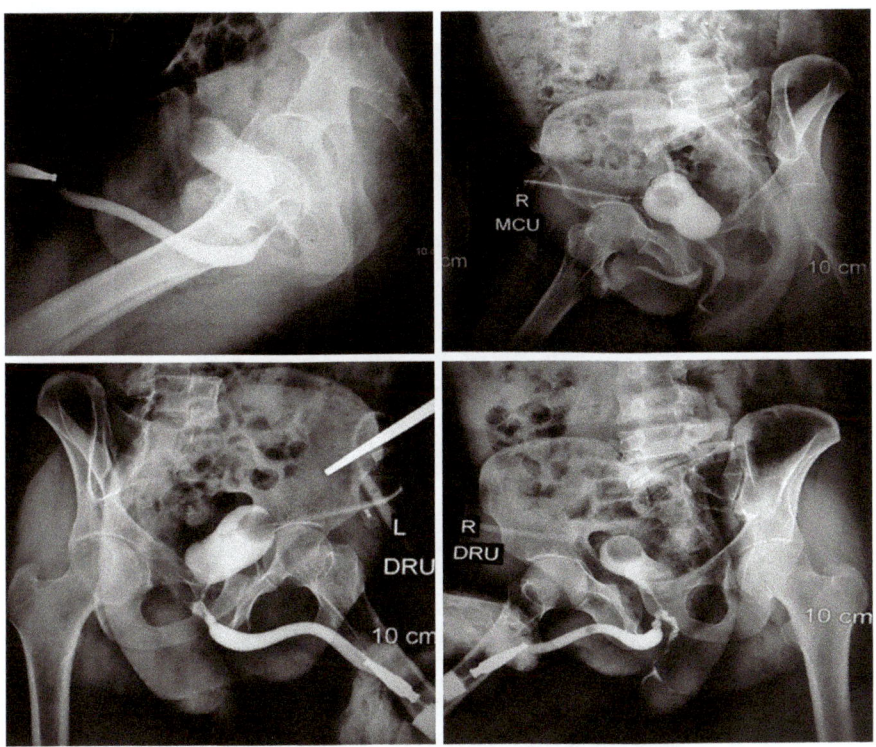

FIG. 22F: The MCU post AKT: Fistula between posterior urethra and anus and stricture at the bulbo-memberanous junction.

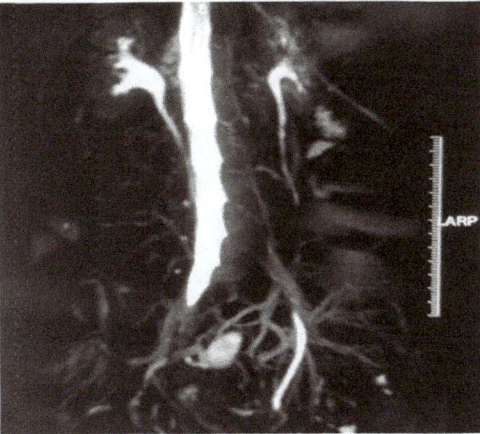

FIG. 22G:

Continued...

Continued...

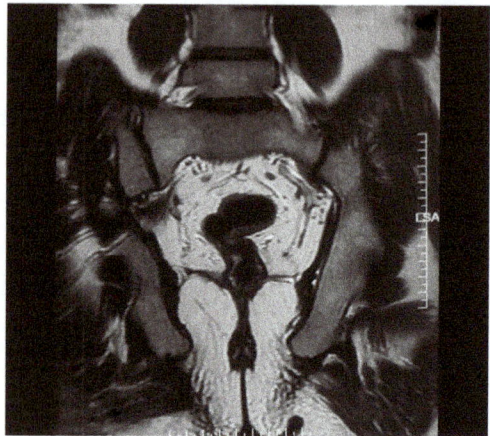

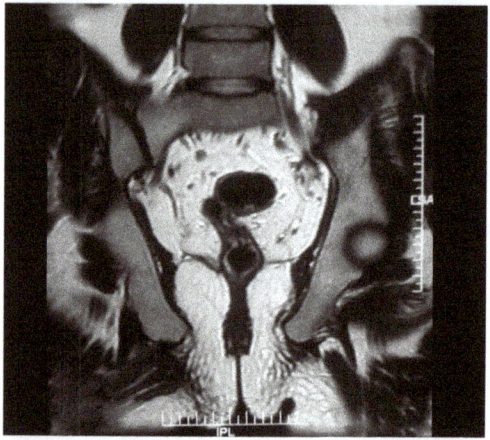

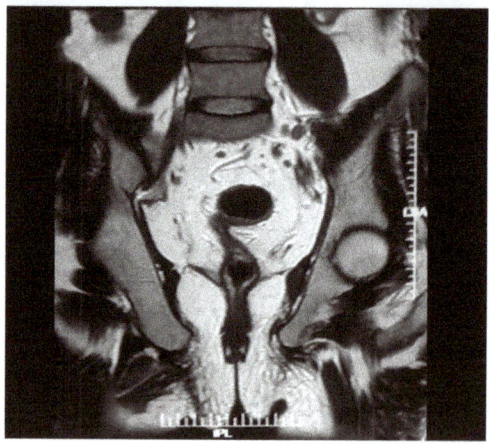

Continued...

Continued...

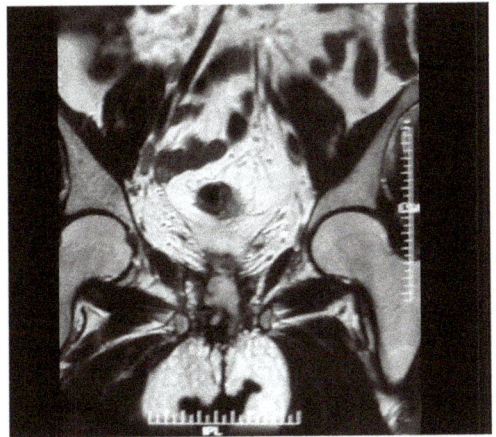

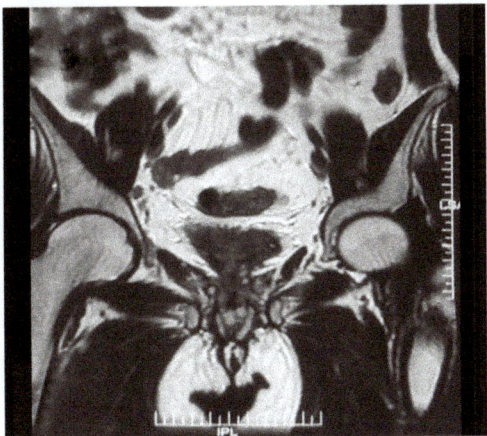

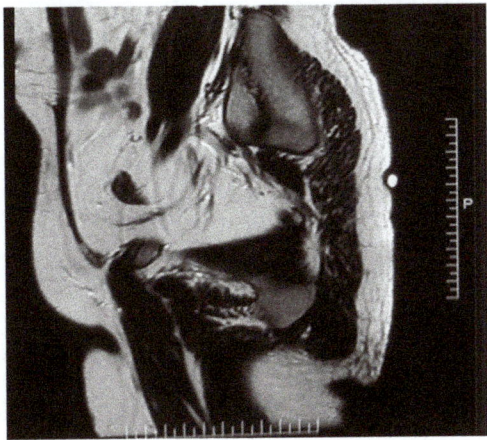

Continued...

Continued...

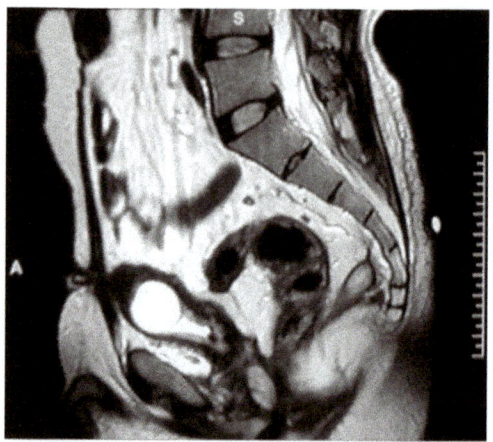

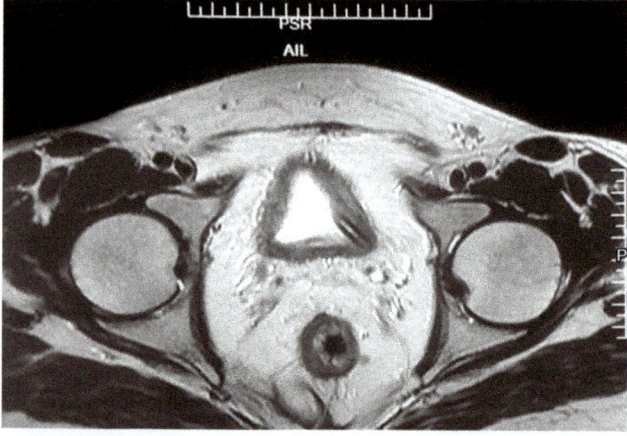

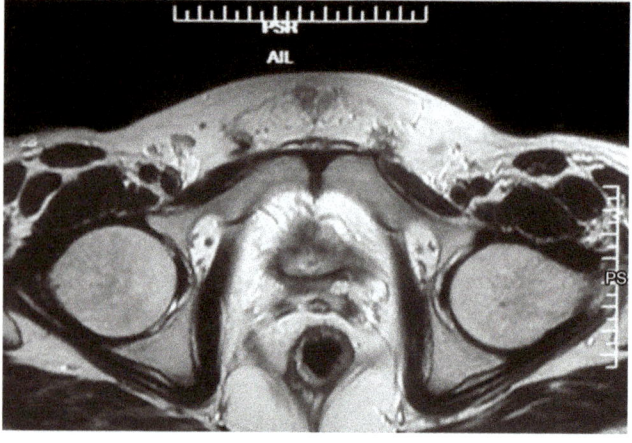

Continued...

Continued...

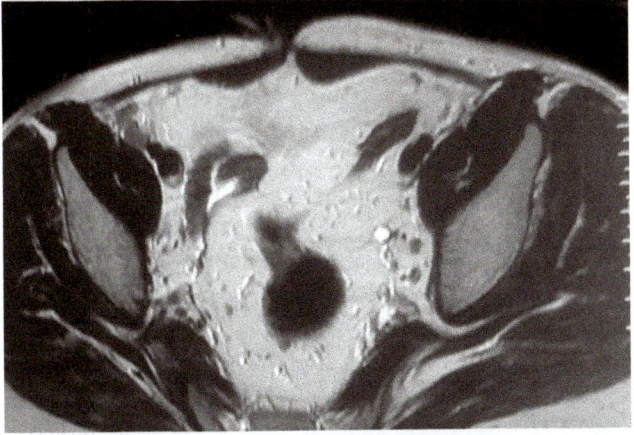

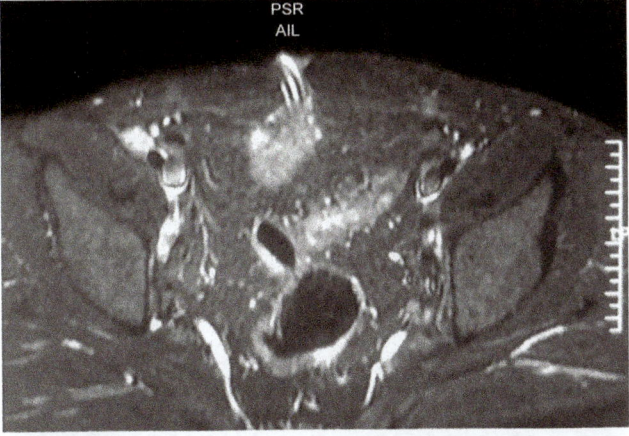

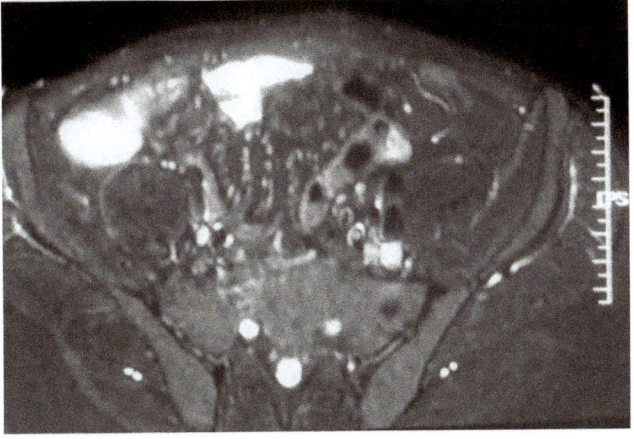

Continued...

Continued...

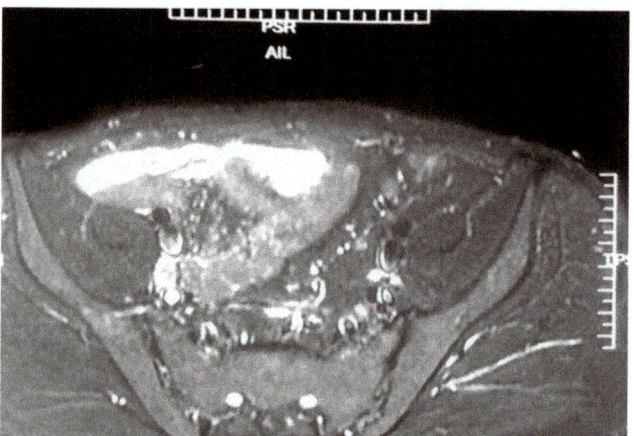

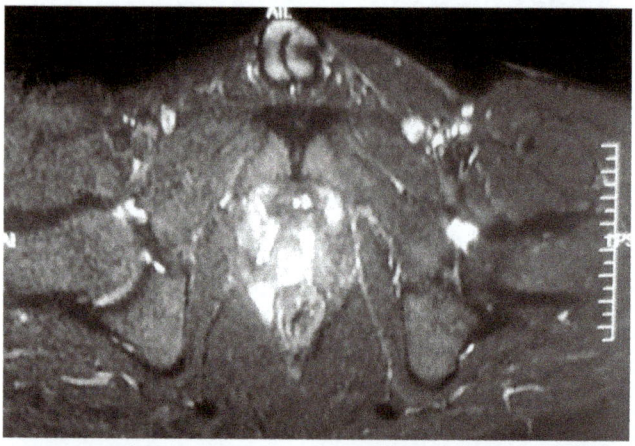

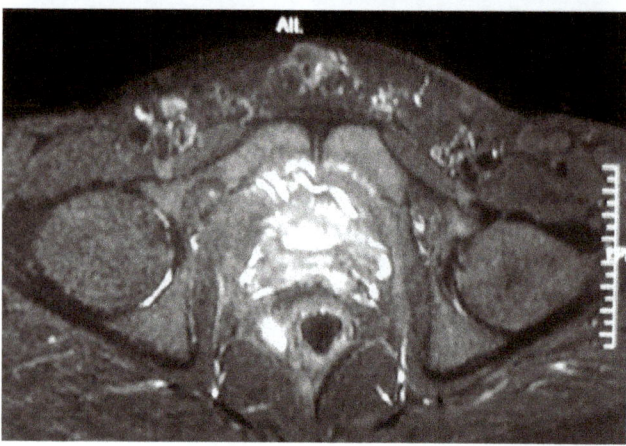

Continued...

Interesting Cases

Continued...

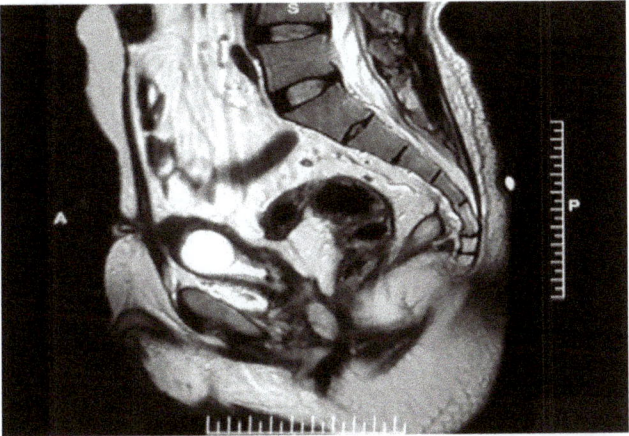

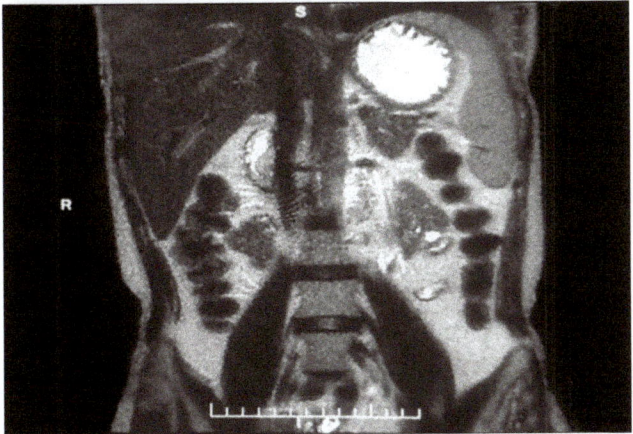

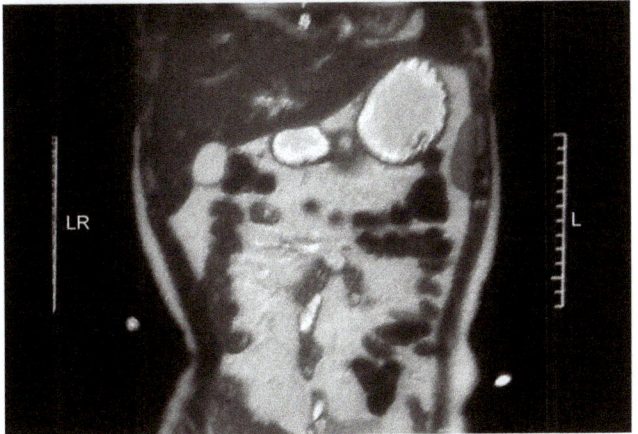

Continued...

Continued...

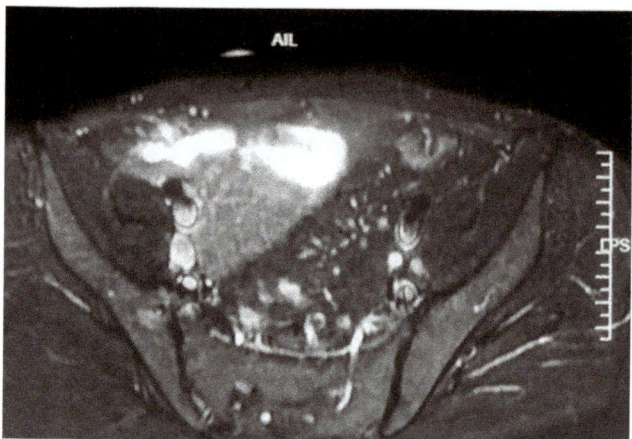

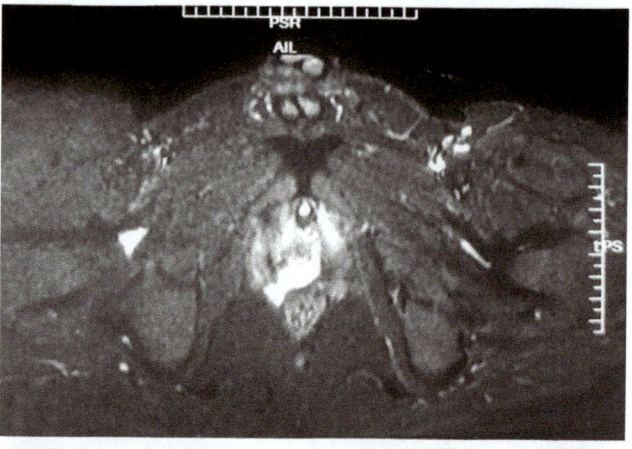

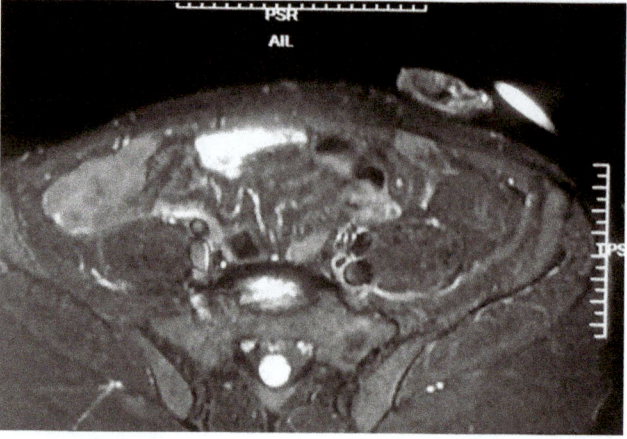

Continued...

Continued...

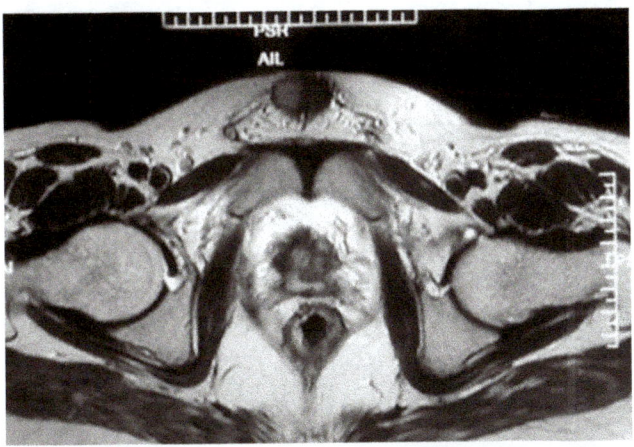

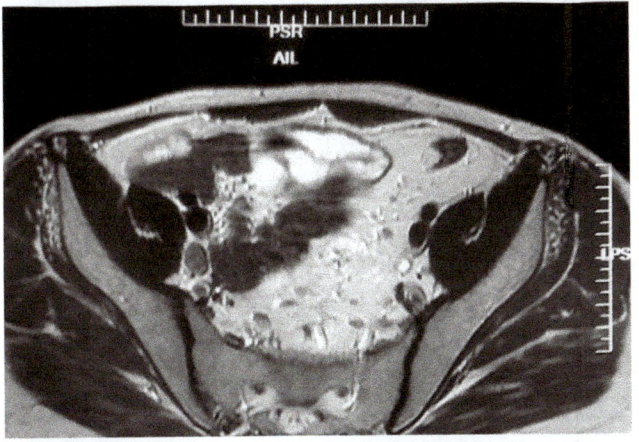

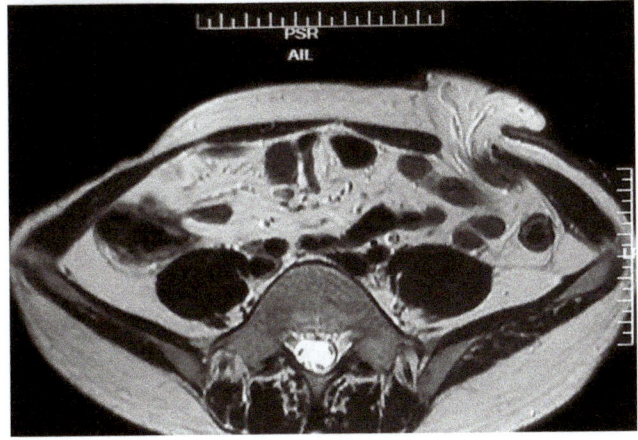

Continued...

Continued...

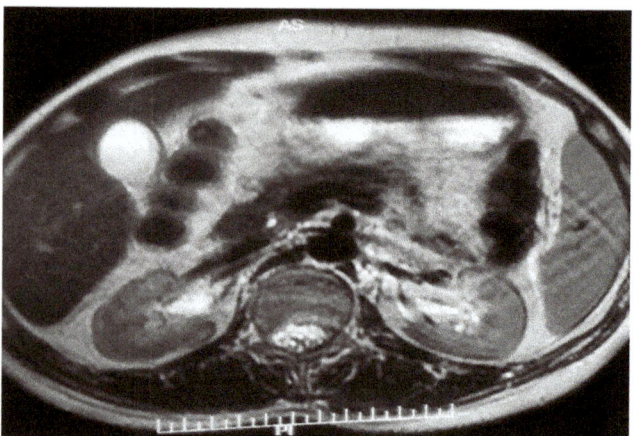

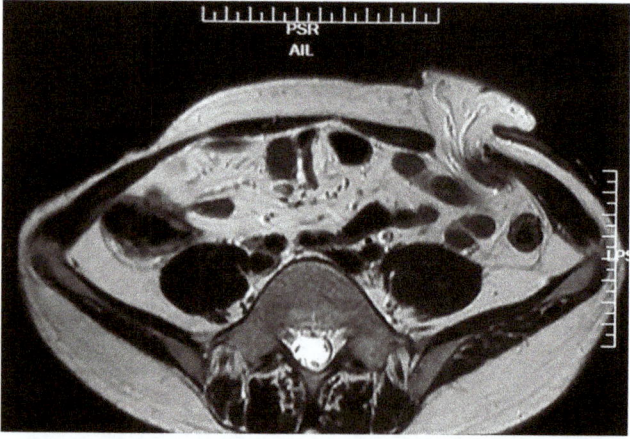

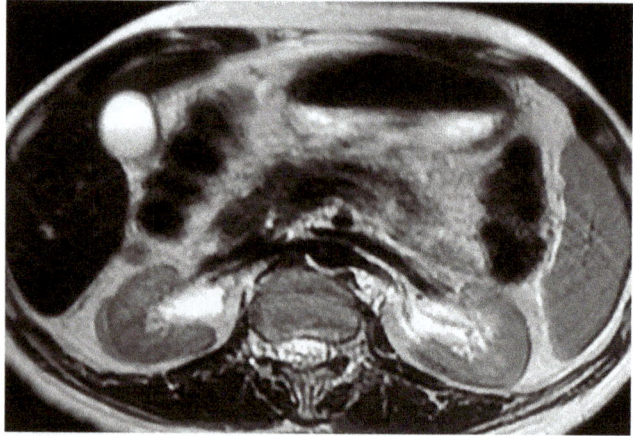

FIG. 22G: MRI pre-AKT.

CASE 23

A 48-year-old man with LUTS for 6 months.

Patient had h/o epididymal abscess of tubercular origin on histopathology elsewhere. Patient has completed AKT last year. Patient has h/o retroviral disease since 5 years and on ART.

Urine analysis: Culture s/o no growth and AFB negative.

Blood investigations: Serum creatinine 1.6 mg/dL and CD4+ count: 384 cells/mm^3.

Chest X-ray: Within normal limits.

USG KUB: Small-sized left kidney with lost CMD and mild dilation of PCS.

RGU: Small contracted bladder with B/L passive vesicoureteral reflux (**Figs. 23 A and B**).

Urethra: Normal.

CT Urogram: **Figures 23C, D, E**.

Right kidney: Normal.

Left kidney: Decreased contrast excretion from left kidney with dilated calyces, infundibular stenosis, shrunken pelvis, and thinned out parenchyma.

Both ureters: Straightening and dilation of both ureters and thickened ureteric walls and evidence of calcification (**Fig. 23E**).

On catheterization: Patient had bladder capacity of only 30 cc.

*DTPA scan (**Fig. 23F**):* Left kidney had differential function of 33% and GFR of 14 m/min with delayed excretion. Right kidney had differential function of 66% and GFR of 28 mL/min.

Left nephrectomy and bladder augmentation was planned. Augmentation by ileo cystoplasty was to be decided intraoperatively if possible as capacity was 30 cc only. Patient was also given an option of augmentation by rat tail anastomosis as he refused an ileal conduit.

He refused surgery but permitted aspiration of urine from left kidney which was sent for prosequencing.

It was positive for tuberculosis with rifampicin resistance.

Patient has been counseled for MDR TB protocol and informed to district TB officer. He is not ready to follow-up.

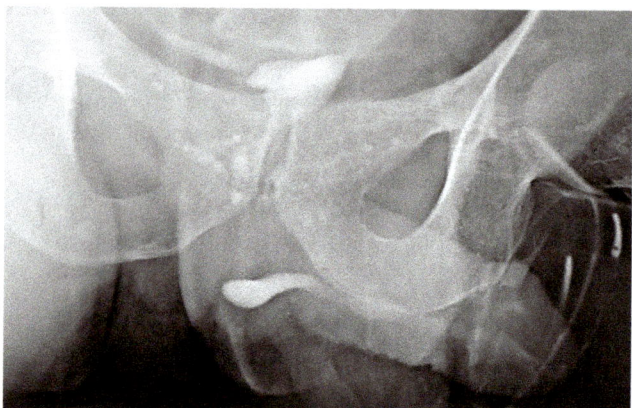

FIG. 23A: Image of RGU showing small capacity bladder with reflux with nonvisualization of posterior urethra.

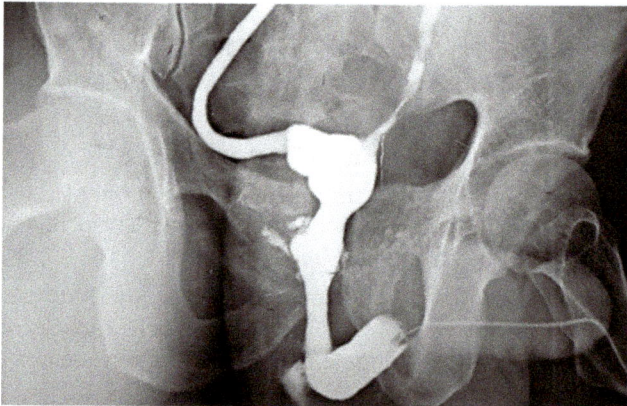

FIG. 23B: Image of MCU showing small capacity bladder with reflux with dilatation of posterior urethra and stricture at bulbomembranous junction.

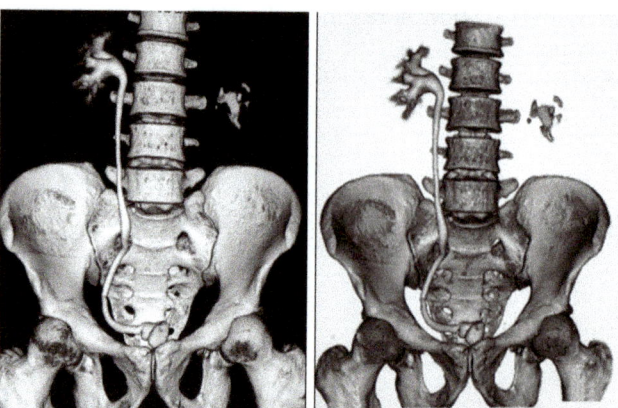

FIG. 23C: Calcified nonfunctioning left kidney with right ureterovesical junction obstruction and small capacity bladder.

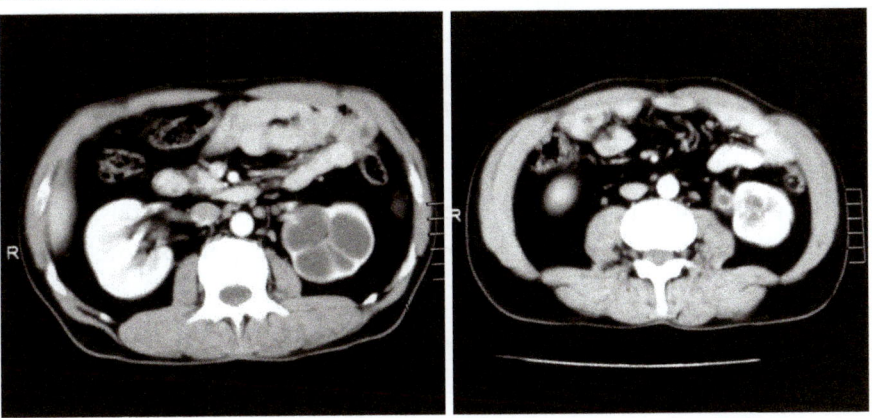

FIG. 23D: Dilated pelvicalyceal system with calcification with thickened upper ureter with nonvisualized pelvis.

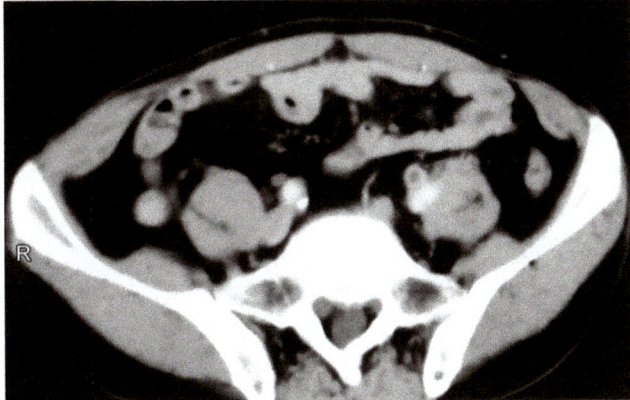

FIG. 23E: Bilateral thickened ureters with calcification.

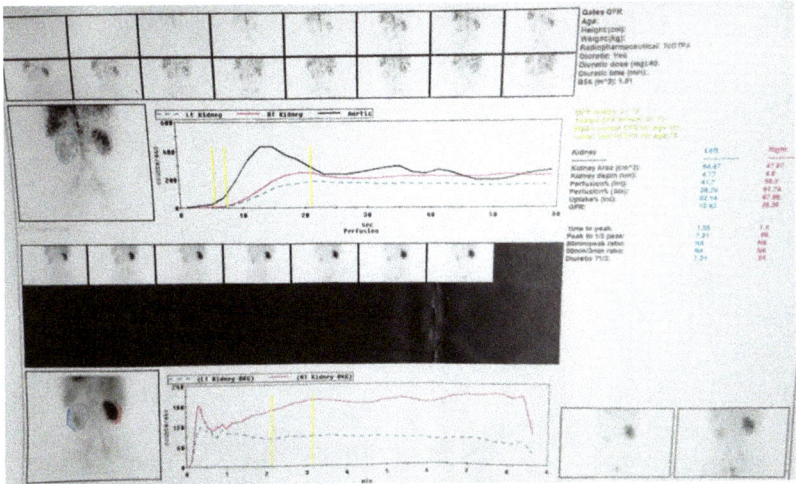

FIG. 23F: Images of DTPA scan.

CASE 24

A 19-year-old female presented with h/o right open pyelolithotomy done 12 years back. Patient had a sinus at surgical site (**Fig. 24A**). Tract excision was done twice in 2009 and 2016. HPE s/o tubercular granulation tissue both times. Patient received AKT twice once for 6 months and second time for 1 year.

At present patient again presented with persistent discharge from the sinus.

On examination: Watery discharge from sinus opening near the previous pyelolithotomy incision.

Investigations

Urine R/M: 304 pus cells/hpf, 102 RBCs, rest WNL.

Blood investigations: HB 10.9 WBC count 5,600 creatinine 1.1.

CECT abdomen and pelvis: 01/02/2019.

Right kidney shows paper thin cortex with multiple cortical calcifications with 1.5 cm pelvic calculus.

Right psoas muscle is bulky with ill-defined collection of 1 cc and surrounding fat stranding with e/o communication of collection with overlying skin leading to sinus (**Figs. 24B and C**).

Left kidney, ureter and bladder normal (**Fig. 24D**).

Urine AFB: 5 days—negative (19/03/2019–24/03/2019).

DTPA scan 27/03/2019 s/o: Non visualized right kidney.

Left kidney: GFR 53.21.

Time to peak: 2.27 min.

Peak to half peak: 7.75 min.

Treatment: Patient underwent open nephrectomy and sinus tract excision (**Figs. 24E and F**).

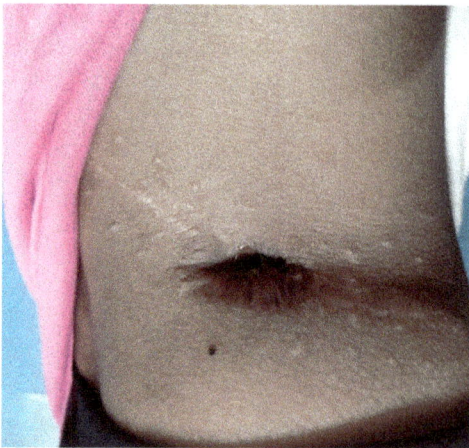

FIG. 24A: Image of sinus.

Interesting Cases

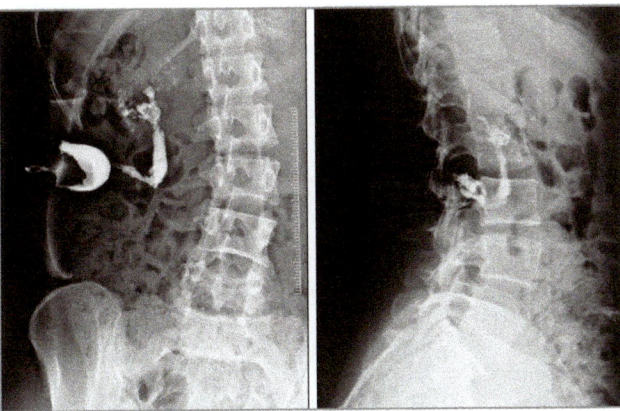

FIG. 24B: Sinogram showing calcified kidney.

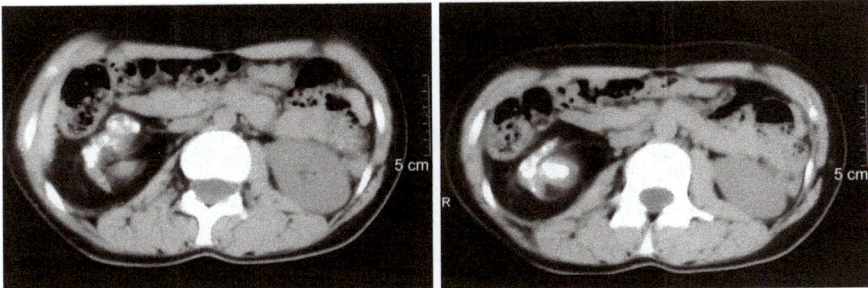

FIG. 24C: Plain CT scan showing right renal parenchymal calcification.

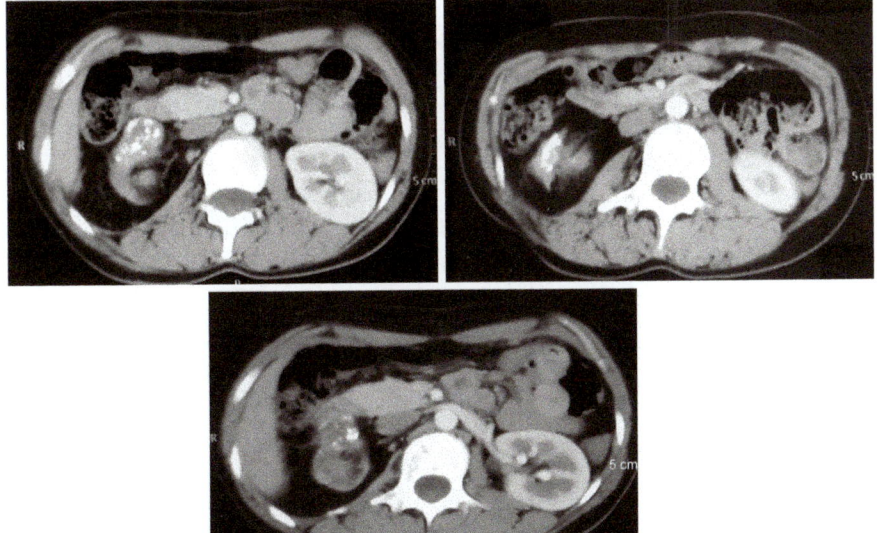

FIG. 24D: Contrast enhanced CT scan showing destroyed right kidney with no function and normal left kidney.

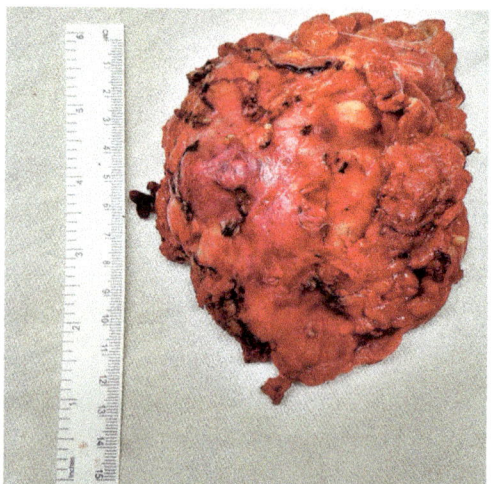

FIG. 24E: Image of external surface of nephrectomy specimen.

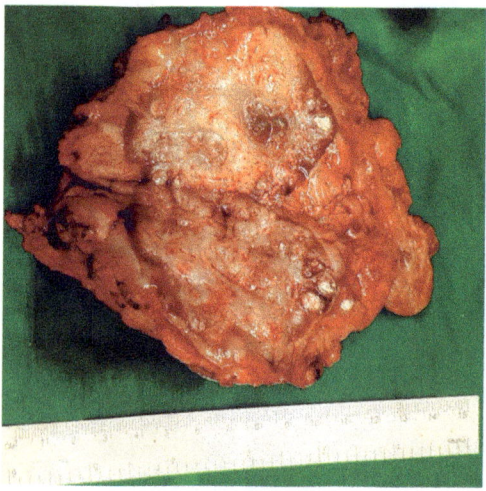

FIG. 24F: Cut surface of kidney showing calcification and caseation.

CASE 25

A 22-year-old male presented with bilateral flank pain since 4 months. He complained of frequency and urgency since 4 months. He had low grade for 4 months. He had a history of pulmonary tuberculosis diagnosed 6 months ago on AKT Category 1.

General examination and routine biochemistry were normal.

Urine AFB: Negative

Urine culture for AFB: Positive

USG KUB:

RK: 9.1 × 3.2 cm.

LK: 9.1 × 4.2 cm.

3.4 × 2.1 cm-sized multilobulated cystic lesion noted in upper pole s/o complex cyst with infective etiology.
Calyectasis noted.

CT urography (Figs. 25A and B):

RK: 11.1 × 5.7 cm.

LK: 10.7 × 5.5 cm. E/o 3.1 × 3.3 × 3.7 cm hypodense peripherally enhancing multiloculated cystic lesion with thin enhancing septa within in upper pole. The lesion has exophytic component abutting adjacent spleen and left psoas muscle. Significant infundibular narrowing and calyectasis are noted.

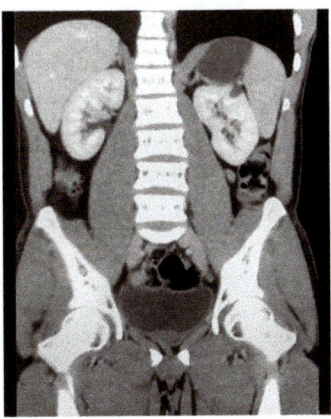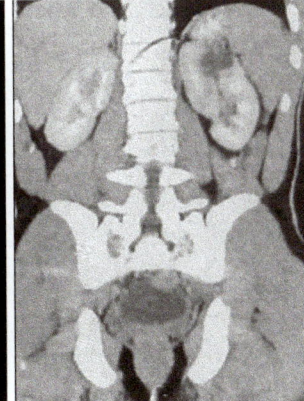

FIG. 25A AND B: CT urography.

CASE 26

An 80-year-old male presented with one episode of painless gross hematuria associated with clots not associated with tissue bits. He had dysuria since 1 month and weight loss since 6 months. No h/o tuberculosis or contact.

General examination and systemic examination were normal.

Investigations

ESR: 136.

Urine AFB: Negative.

Urine GeneXpert: Negative.

X-ray: Left renal area.

USG KUB: Left-sided putty kidney.

Calcification: (**Fig. 26A**)

Left renal parenchyma is near completely replaced with dense chunky lobar calcification (average HU + 700). Residual parenchyma at upper pole (UPPT-4 mm) and midpole (MPPT-3 mm) shows poor nephrogram and no excretion of contrast even on 3 hours delayed scan suggestive of Putty kidney (**Fig. 26B**).

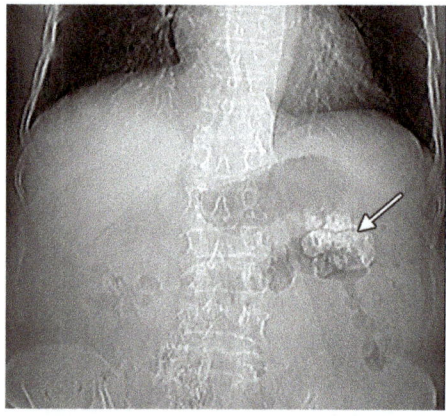

FIG. 26A: Plain X-ray showing dense chunky calcification in region of left kidney.

Interesting Cases 187

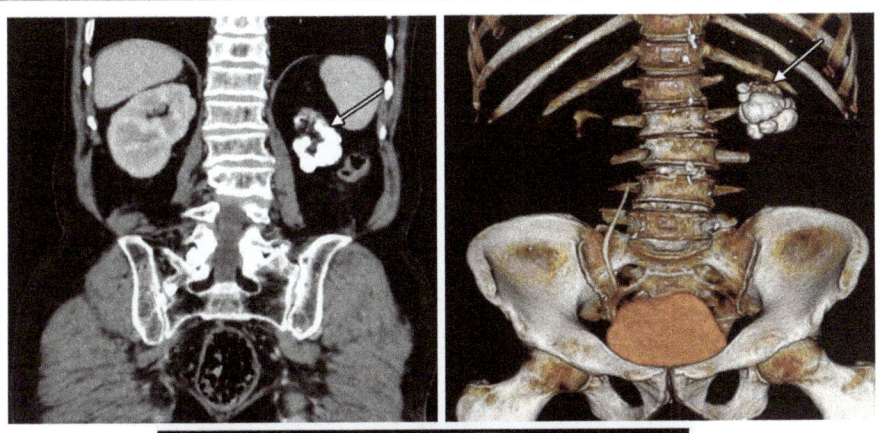

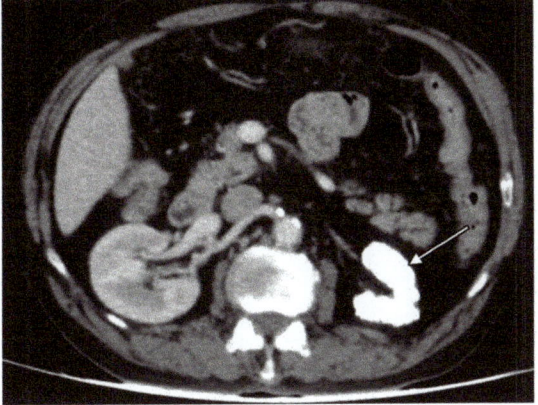

FIG. 26B: CT urography showing normal hypertrophied right kidney with completely calcified left kidney. Patient underwent open nephrectomy.

INDEX

Page numbers followed by *f* refer to figure, *fc* refer to flowchart, and *t* refer to table.

A

Abdomen 156
  plain 52
Abdominal wall, posterior 64*f*, 118*f*
Abscess
  developing 113*f*, 117*f*
  multiple 115*f*, 116*f*, 119*f*
  perinephric 56, 64*f*
  perirenal extension of 118*f*
  thick-walled 117*f*
  tuberculous 82*f*
  wall of 113*f*, 114*f*
Absolute neutrophils count 23
Acid-fast bacilli 38*f*, 45, 49
Adherence monitoring system, mobile-based 3
Adnexa, oblique scan of 89*f*
Airborne infection control 12
Air-filled tract 74
Alanine aminotransferase 23
Amenorrhea 87
Amikacin 22, 47, 94
Aminosalicylic acid 94
Amoxicillin 9, 9*f*, 22
Anal canal 77*f*
Anorexia 98, 155
Antegrade nephrostogram 107*f*
Anti-Koch treatment 47
Antiretroviral therapy 10
Antitubercular therapy 6
Anti-tuberculosis drugs 22*t*
  classes of 21
  newer 14, 21
Anti-tuberculous
  first-line drugs 94*t*
  second-line drugs 94*t*
Appetite, decreased 114
Ascites 87
Aspartate aminotransferase 23
Asymmetric caliectasis 69*f*
Augmentation cystoplasty 108
Autonephrectomy 56, 74*f*
Autopsy 39

B

Bacillus Calmette-Guérin vaccine 13
Bacterial pyelonephritis, acute 54
Bacteriological monitoring 27
Balloon dilatation 95
Bedaquiline 14, 22, 23, 94
Bladder 99, 102
  augmentation 102, 107
  MCU-full 135*f*
  MCU-small 156*f*
  small
    capacity 139*f*, 142*f*, 180*f*
    contracted 157*f*
  surgery 96
  thickened 120*f*, 157*f*, 165*f*
    wall of 123*f*, 132*f*, 146*f*
  tuberculosis of 41
  urine 46
Boari flap 106
Bowel segment 102
Brucellosis 43
Buccal mucosa 108*f*
Bulbar urethra 120*f*
Bulbomemberanous junction 169*f*, 180*f*

C

Calcified kidney 95, 183*f*
Calcium, milk of 67*f*
Calicorrhaphy 102
Calyceal infundibular stenosis, left superior 149*f*
Calyces
  lower 69*f*
  mucosal thickening of 64*f*
  thick-walled 122*f*
Calyectasis, evaluation of 57
Calyx
  focal caliectasis of minor 68*f*
  lower pole 62*f*
  middle 69*f*
  selectively, left upper 162*f*
Capreomycin 22, 94
Caseating granulomas, multiple 39*f*

Caseous necrosis 37
  large area of 37f
Catholic Bishops' conference 11
Catholic Church healthcare facilities 11
Cavernotomy 100
Central caseous necrosis 36f, 37
Central tuberculosis division 4
Cerebrospinal fluid 7
Chemotherapy 98
Cilastatin 22
Clarithromycin 9, 94
Clavulanate 22
Clavulanic acid 9
Clofazimine 9, 9f, 22
Complete blood count 92
Computed tomography scan 54
Co-trimoxazole preventive therapy 10
Crohn's disease 102
CT urography 185, 185f, 187f
Cutaneous fistula 167f
Cycloserine 9, 22, 94
Cystectomy 96
Cystoplasty, complications of 108

D

Delamanid 22
Dense chunky calcification 186f
Dense perinephric adhesions 112
Deoxyribonucleic acid 47
Diabetes 93
  mellitus 10, 48
Diethylenetriamine pentaacetate 104
  scan 179, 181f, 182
Diffusion-weighted imaging 57
Directly observed treatment short-course 33
  strategy 1
Disseminated infection 39
Distorted calyces 131f
Distorted pelvicalyceal system 131f
Distorting calyx 62f
District Tuberculosis Center 4, 19
District Tuberculosis Officer 4
DMSA renogram 134, 140
Dormant bacteria 92
Double J stent 99
Drug-resistance
  diagnostic technology choice 18
  tests 17
Drug-resistant tuberculosis 1, 20
  center 16
  classification of 14, 15
  diagnostic algorithm guidelines 2019 20fc
  management of 14, 24, 28, 29
    programmatic 8, 9, 15, 20

Drug-susceptibility testing 17, 20, 29
  methods for 14, 16
Drugs, new grouping of 22
Duodenum repair 112
Duodenum 55
Dystrophic calcifications 75f
Dysuria 186

E

Ectopia, cross-fused 144f
Eggshell calcification 122f
Ejaculatory ducts 78f, 79f
Endometrial osseous metaplasia 87
Endometrial polyp 87
Endometrial tuberculosis 87
Endometrium 90f, 91f
  irregular contour of 87
E-NIKSHAY 32
  role of 33
Epididymal cysts, multiple 79f
Epididymal tuberculosis 74
Epididymis 75, 78f, 79f, 84
  head of 81f
  tail of 81f-83f
  tuberculosis of 42
  tuberculous lesion of tail of 82f
Epithelioid cells 36
Epithelioid granuloma 36, 36f
  multiple 43
Epithelioid macrophages 37
Escherichia coli 43, 112
Ethambutol 9, 22, 47, 94
Ethionamide 9, 22, 94
Ethylene dicysteine 104
Extensive drug resistance 6, 15
Extensively drug-resistant tuberculosis,
  diagnosis of 9
Extrapulmonary tuberculosis, sequelae of 7

F

Fallopian tube 84, 90f
  floating 87
Fibrotic bladder 109f
Fibrous tissue 37
First-line line probe assay 20
Fistulas 55
  multiple 166f
  persistent 95
  rectal opening of 167f
Flank pain, bilateral 185
Fluid distended fallopian tube,
  thick-walled 90f
Fluid samples 46
Fluoroquinolone 20, 22

Focal calyectasis 147
Focal nodular heterogeneous lesion 83*f*
Food and Drug Administration 21
Fungal infections 36, 40

G

Gas-filled fistulous tract 77*f*
Gatifloxacin 22
GeneXpert 50
    detection 140
Genital surgery 97
Genital tract
    male 74
    tuberculosis, female 84
Genitourinary physicians and surgeons 110
Genitourinary tract 36, 38
Genitourinary tuberculosis 14, 43, 45, 48,
    52, 93
    diagnosis of 45, 47, 48
    disease 93
    management of 45
    sample collection for 45
Gerota's fascia 57, 114*f*
Giant hydrocalyx 103
Gömöri methenamine silver 42
Granuloma 36*f*, 37, 57
    healing of 75*f*
    multiple 126
        noncaseating 40*f*
    resection 41
Granulomatous disease, types of 36
Granulomatous infection 134
Granulomatous inflammation 40, 41
Granulomatous orchitis 43
Granulomatous prostatitis, nonspecific 42
Growth indicator tube 46

H

Heart failure 23
Hematological investigations 118
Hematuria 96, 140
Heminephrectomy 100, 104
Hemoglobin 23
Hepatitis
    B 92
    C 92
Heterogeneous hypoechoic
    nodules 75
    texture 84*f*
High-resolution ultrasonography 60, 66*f*
Hilar lymph nodes 122*f*
Histoplasma capsulatum 43
Homogeneous hypoechoic
    epididymis, diffusely enlarged 81*f*
    nodules 75

Homogenous consolidation, large 141*f*
Horse shoe kidney 144*f*
Human immunodeficiency virus 1, 9, 43,
    48, 92
    testing 32
Hydrocalycosis, left superior 149*f*
Hydrocele 84*f*
    chronic 83*f*
Hydronephrosis 66, 66*f*
    evaluation of 57
    left 157*f*
    right 139*f*
        moderate 134*f*, 135*f*
    with left upper ureteric 146*f*
Hydronephrotic kidney 73*f*
    calcified walls of 74*f*
    right 152*f*
Hydrosalpinx 90*f*
Hydroureteronephrosis
    bilateral 129*f*
    proximal 146*f*, 148*f*
Hypodensities, multiple 127*f*
Hypoechoic epididymis 80*f*
Hypoechoic masses, multiple 160*f*
Hypoechoic nodules, multiple small 84*f*
Hypokalemia 23, 107
Hysteroscopic biopsy 87

I

Idiopathic granulomatous orchitis 43
Ileal conduits 109
Ileocalicostomy 101*f*
Imipenem 22
Immune reconstitution inflammatory
    syndrome 27
Indian Academy of Pediatrics 10
Infection control measures 14, 33
Infundibular stenosis 149*f*
    multiple 136*f*
Infundibuloplasty 101*f*, 104
Infundibulum
    fibrosis of 68*f*
    surgery for 96
Injectable agents, second-line 22
Institute of Leprosy and other Mycobacterial
    Diseases 4
Intensive case finding 2
Interstitial nephritis 39
    drug-induced 40
Intestine, distal small 158
Intrarenal pelvis 164*f*
Intravenous pyelogram 53
    nephrogram phase of 149*f*
Intravenous pyelography 105*f*, 140, 142*f*, 143,
    148, 150*f*, 153, 156
    normal 154*f*

Intravenous urography 52, 104
Irritative voiding symptoms 84
Isoniazid 6, 9, 47, 94
    high-dose 9f, 22
    preventive therapy 10, 13

J

Jan Dhan Yojana 3
Joint Secretary of Health 4

K

Kanamycin 22, 94
Kaplan-Meier survival estimator 111
Kerr's kink 66
Kidney 38, 120f
    cement 40
    coronal scan of 64f, 65f, 67f, 69f, 70f
    cut surface of 184f
    disease epidemiology collaboration, chronic 104
    extensive calcification of 73f
    high-resolution ultrasonography image of 60f-63f
    interstitium of 40f
    material inside 138
    nonfunctioning 95
    nonvisualization of 56
    transverse scan of 64f, 65f, 70f
    tuberculosis of 38, 39f
    underwent nephrectomy 106
Koch's contact 133, 151, 153

L

Langhans giant cells 36, 37
Langhans type 37f
Laparoscopic nephrectomy 95
Laparotomy, exploratory 158
Latent tuberculosis infection treatment 12
Left kidney 131f, 144f, 179
    lower pole of 148f
    nonfunctioning 139f, 180f
    normal 183f
    parenchymal calcification in 134f, 135f
    region of 186f
    upper pole of 67f
Left lower ureter 132f
    stricture 121f, 132f, 142f
Left ureteric
    calculus 145, 145f
    dilatation 131f
    wall calcification 123f
Leprosy 36, 43
Leukemia, acute 13
Levofloxacin 9, 22, 94

Line probe assay 9, 17
Linezolid 9, 9f, 22, 94
Lipoarabinomannan 51
Lithuria 140
Liver 55
    disease, chronic 58
    function test 92
Lobar caseation 56
Lung field, right 141f
Lymph nodes 39f
    retroperitoneal 120f
Lymphadenopathy, abdominal 144f
Lymphocytes 37

M

Magnetic resonance urography 57
Malaria 11
Mass lesion 39
MCU/RGU prostatic-rectal fistula 167f
MCU-bilateral reflux 164f
MCU-bladder 160f
Medical Officer-Tuberculosis Control 4
Medically resistant hypertension 95
Medication event reminder monitor system 30
Medullary cavity
    irregular 63f
    large 62f
Meropenem 22
Micturating cystogram 130f
Micturating cystourethrogram 132f, 135, 139, 142, 155
Midureter
    high-resolution ultrasonography image of 67f
    oblique scan of 71f
Midureteric strictures, bilateral 137f
Miliary tuberculosis 5
Millennium development goal 2
Minimally invasive management 95
Moxifloxacin 9, 22, 94
Multidetector computed tomography 54
Multidrug-resistant
    pulmonary tuberculosis 25
    tuberculosis 22
        diagnosis of 9
Multinucleated giant cells 37f
Multiple drug therapy 92
Mycobacteria 38, 39
    infections, atypical 56
Mycobacterium 47
    avium-intracellulare 38
    smegmatis 49
    tuberculosis 5, 17, 45, 50, 92, 140
Mycolic acid 38

N

Nadir serum creatinine 108
Narrow pelvis, parenchymal calcification
    with 135*f*
National AIDS Control Programme 2
National Expert Technical Working Group 15
National Framework for Joint TB-HIV
    Collaborative Activities 2, 10
National Health Mission 2
National Institute for Research in
    Tuberculosis 4
National Japanese Leprosy Mission for Asia 4
National Reference Laboratory 8
National Strategic Plan for Tuberculosis
    Elimination 2
National Technical Working Group 11
National Tuberculosis Control Programme
    free of cost 47
    objectives of revised 33
    revised 1, 10, 14, 15, 29, 34
National Tuberculosis Institute 4
National Tuberculosis Programme 1
    surveillance system 32
Nausea 114
Nephrectomy 95, 98
    after 139*f*
    before 139*f*
    partial 100, 101*f*, 104
    specimen 184*f*
Nephrocutaneous fistula 62
Nephrostogram 101*f*
Nephrotic syndrome 13
Newer information and communication
    technology solutions 30
NIKSHAY 3, 14, 32
    scheme 92
Nocturia 96
Nodular lesion 154*f*
Nucleic acid
    amplification test 17, 50
        cartridge based 7, 20, 47, 92

O

Omental flap 108*f*
Orchidectomy 97
Orthotopic bladder 102
Orthotopic substitution 109

P

P-aminosalicylic acid 22
Papillary necrosis 69
Para-aminosalicylic acid 9
Parenchyma 55, 152*f*
Parenchymal calcification 131*f*, 145*f*, 152*f*, 164*f*
    left 124*f*

Parenchymal cavity 60, 64*f*
    large irregular 61*f*
    multiple 70*f*
Parenchymal cyst, small 67*f*
Parenchymal mass 60*f*, 61*f*
Parenchymal nodules 54
Parenchymal tuberculomas 53
Parietal wall 87
Paucibacillary disease 45
Pelvic brim 148*f*
    level of 71*f*
Pelvic infundibular strictures 56
Pelvic stricture 54, 69*f*, 96
Pelvic tuberculosis, dry type of 90*f*
Pelvicalyceal anatomy of kidney 101*f*
Pelvicalyceal system 53, 96, 127
    dilated 181*f*
        left 156*f*
    left 156
    normal 137*f*, 168*f*
        right 156*f*
    right 164*f*
        distorted 146*f*
Pelvis 96, 156
    left small 136*f*
    mucosal thickening of 64*f*
    nonvisualized 181*f*
    sagittal scan of 88*f*
    tuberculosis of 41
Pelviureteric junction 64, 66, 105*f*
    obstruction, lower moiety 144*f*
    stenosis of 66*f*
Penis, ventral surface of 154*f*
Percutaneous nephrostomy 95, 99, 105*f*, 106,
    109
    obstruction 121, 121*f*, 132, 132*f*, 133, 133*f*,
        136, 136*f*, 139, 142
Perinephric fat stranding 57, 112, 113*f*, 114*f*
Periodic acid-Schiff 42
Periodic ureteric dilatation 103
Peripheral Health Institution 5, 18
Perirenal fat stranding 117*f*
Peritoneum, thickening of 88*f*
Phantom calyx, left upper 162*f*
Phenotypic drug susceptibility testing, growth-
    based 17
Plasma cells 37
Pleura 55
Pleural fluid adenosine deaminase activity 7
Polymerase chain reaction 6, 47, 50
Post-ileocalicostomy nephrostogram 102*f*
Pott's spine, old healed 122*f*
Prostate 74, 86*f*, 99, 102
    axial scan of 76*f*, 77*f*
    gland 74
    longitudinal scan of 76*f*

tuberculosis of 41
   involvement of 41
Prostatectomy 166
Prostatic architecture, destroyed 168*f*
Prostatic substitution 102
Prothionamide 22
Pseudomonas aeruginosa 133, 140
Pseudotumor 39
Psoas
   abscess 114*f*
     right 119*f*
   and adjacent abdominal wall 116*f*
   involvement of 114*f*
   muscle 127*f*
     left 185
Public finance management system 3
Pulmonary Koch's 133, 151, 153
Pulmonary tuberculosis 5, 14, 48
   active 141*f*
   drug-sensitive 25
   mono-drug resistant 26
   poly-drug resistant 26
Punctuate calcification 56
Putty kidney 40, 53, 69, 73*f*, 186
   left 125*f*
Putty-like calcification 68
Pyelo fistulae 55
Pyelography, retrograde 53
Pyelolysis 101*f*, 104
Pyelonephritis 39, 107
Pyeloureteric anastomosis 102
Pyogenic epididymo orchitis 43
Pyonephrosis 40, 70*f*
Pyosalpingitis 87
Pyrazinamide 22, 92, 94

Q

QT syndrome, long 23

R

Radionucleotide scintigraphy 106
Rat tail anastomosis 97
Reconstructive surgery 99, 103
Reconstructive surgical procedures 99
   indications for 100
Regional Medical Research Centre 4
Renal abscess 55, 64*f*, 117*f*
Renal area, coronal scan of 73*f*, 74*f*
Renal calcification, left 122*f*
Renal calculus, right multiple 146*f*
Renal disease, end-stage 52
Renal failure, chronic 106
Renal fistulae 55
Renal function 99
   global 102

   preservation of 99, 110
   test 92
Renal infundibuloplasty 102
Renal lobes 98
Renal nuclear scintigraphy 104
Renal parenchyma 37*f*, 54, 57, 60
   calcification, left 122*f*
   left 186
Renal pelvis 69*f*
   dilatation 66
   extensive calcification of wall of 73*f*
   kinking of 70*f*
Renal tuberculosis, localized 39
Renal unit
   damage, obstruction related 98
   function
     assessment 111
     opposite 111
Renocutaneous fistula 55
Respiratory infections, acute 12
Rifabutin 94
Rifampicin 6, 47, 50
Rifampin 94
Right kidney 124*f*, 144*f*
   calcified lower pole of 120*f*
   destroyed 183*f*
   middle pole of 152*f*
   nonfunctioning 120*f*
   nonvisualized 142*f*
   normal
     functioning 144*f*
     hypertrophied 187*f*
Right renal
   abscess 127*f*
   calculus 145*f*
   parenchyma 125*f*, 127*f*
     calcification 183*f*
   pelvis 164*f*

S

Sarcoidosis 36, 40
Scarred cavity 87
Scars 166*f*
Scrotal abscess formation 42
Scrotum
   empty 166*f*
   scan of 83*f*
Seminal vesicle 74, 84, 85*f*, 86*f*
   tuberculosis of 80
Senior Tuberculosis Laboratory Supervisor 4
Senior Tuberculosis Treatment Supervisor 4
Serum
   creatinine 109, 134, 166
     continues 164
   electrolytes 134, 152

Shrunken bladder, small 139f
Shrunken kidney, left 125f
Sinus 182f
   tract 55, 128f
      thick-walled 128f
Sonolucent tract 63f
Speleotomy 100, 103
   procedure 100f
Spermatic cord 85f
State tuberculosis cells 4
State Tuberculosis Officer 4
State tuberculosis training and demonstration centre 4
Status simultaneous ureteropyelostomy 105f
Steroids, role of 93
Streptomycin 22, 47, 94
Stress incontinence 109
Synechia 87, 90f
Syphilis 36
Systemic infection 98

T

Terizidone 22
Testicular tuberculosis 74
Testis 75, 80, 84f
   diffusely enlarged 84f
   enlarged 84f
   enlargement of 79
   scan of 79f
   tuberculosis of 42
Thiacetazone 9
Thioacetazone 22
Tifampicin-susceptible tuberculosis 20
Tissue 92
   samples 46
Transplanted kidney, tuberculosis in 58
Transport box, technical specifications of 19f
Transureteroureterostomies 106
Transurethral resection 108
Treponema pallidum 42
Trigone area, Mucosal thickening of 71f
TRUS-prostate gland measures 160f
Tubercular urethral involvement 109
Tuberculoma, wall of 124f
Tuberculosis 9-11, 20, 36, 41, 43, 45, 74, 85f, 89f, 90f, 96, 98, 136
   adhesive type 87
   algorithm, integrated drug-resistant 14, 19, 21fc, 24
   childhood 10
   culture 50
   diagnosis of 47
      molecular approaches for 47
   disease 1
   dry type 87
   epidemiology 1
   etiology 119
   extrapulmonary 5, 20, 27, 48
   gastrointestinal 96
   granulomas 52
   infection 12
   pathology of 36
   pediatric 27
   poly-drug resistant 15
   recurrent 6
   rifampicin
      resistant 15, 20, 22
      susceptible 20
   sputum 140
   strictures 95
   treatment of 92
      drug-resistant 14, 21
      extensively drug-resistant 9
      history of 5
      multidrug-resistant 9
   unit level 4
   wet type 87
Tuberculous contracture 108
Tuberculous epididymitis 42, 74, 80f
Tuberculous epididymo-orchitis 43f
Tuberculous granulomatous interstitial nephritis 40f
Tuberculous interstitial nephritis 40
Tuberculous orchitis, isolated 42
Tuberculous perinephric abscess 64f
Tuberculous pyelonephritis 40
Tuberculous ulceration 95
Tubes, enlargement of 87
Tubo-ovarian abscess 89f
   formation 87
Tunica vaginalis, calcification of 83f

U

Ulcerative colitis 102
Unhealthy bladder 158f
Upper calyx 69f
Upper ureteric stricture
   buccal mucosa augmentation of 107
   repair 108f
Ureter 95, 156f
   color Doppler image of 71f
   dilated 128f, 146f
      left 119f
      proximal 66f, 71f
      thickened right 125f
   ileal
      replacement of 102
      substitution of 107
   narrow, right lower 156f
   oblique scan of 71f

right 148*f*
  lower 155
  thick 116*f*
    walled distal 146*f*
  tuberculosis of 41
  with thick walls, dilated right 124*f*
Ureteral urine samples 147
Ureteric calcification, bilateral 137*f*
Ureteric dilatation 103
  efficacy of 103
  mild 142*f*
Ureteric procedures, lower 104
Ureteric reimplant 105*f*, 106
  surgical procedures of 106
Ureteric stricture 96
  bilateral 138*f*
  buccal mucosal grafting augmentation of 102
  lower 139*f*
  multiple left 133*f*
  right distal 136*f*
Ureteric wall calcification and thickening 117*f*
Ureterocalicostomy 96, 102, 105, 106
Ureterogram, retrograde 108*f*
Ureteroneocystostomy 102, 106
Ureteropyelostomy 104
Ureteroureterostomy 106
Ureterovesical junction 95
  obstruction, right 180*f*
Ureters with calcification, bilateral thickened 181*f*
Urethra 99
  and anus, posterior 169*f*
  gas outlining 77*f*
  nonvisualization of posterior 180*f*
  posterior 180*f*
  procedures for 103
Urethral fistula excision 166
Urethral stricture 109
Urethroplasty 103, 109
Urinary bladder 68, 72*f*, 73*f*, 86*f*
  and vagina 156*f*
  fibrosis of walls of 73*f*
  oblique scan of 71*f*
  small capacity 142*f*
  transverse scan of 72*f*
Urinary conduits, obstruction of 98
Urinary tuberculosis 49, 49*t*, 60, 69, 98, 110
  context of 98
  sonographic features of 60
Urine
  acid-fast staining 49
  analysis 179
  collection, method of 45
  samples 45
Urodynamic study 143
Uterus, longitudinal scan of 91*f*

V

Vagina, contrast in 157*f*
Vas deferens 86*f*
  hypoechoic mass of 85*f*
Vasa deferentia 80
Vesicoureteric junction 130*f*
  obstruction 129*f*
  right 125*f*
  stricture 133*f*, 139*f*
    left 142*f*
Vesicoureteric reflux 71*f*
  bilateral 132*f*
Vesicourethral anastomosis 166
Vesicovaginal fistula 96
  large 158*f*
Vomiting 114

W

Weight loss 98
World Health Organization 1
World Health Organization Global Tuberculosis Report 8

X

Xanthogranulomatous pyelonephritis 40

Z

Ziehl-Neelsen
  smear 49
  stain 38, 38*f*, 42, 46

EU GSPR Authorised Reprsentative
Logos Europe, 9 rue Nicolas Poussin
1700, La Rochelle, France
Phone: +33 (0) 6 67 93 73 78
E-mail: contact@logoseurope.eu

www.ingramcontent.com/pod-product-compliance
Ingram Content Group UK Ltd.
Pitfield, Milton Keynes, MK11 3LW, UK
UKHW050427150426
5217IPUK00019B/1273